I0758597

Comparing the Mediterranean Diet and the Blue Zone Diet

The Mediterranean diet is nothing new. It's been praised for years as a heart-healthy way to eat, but with new research, and continued support of the Blue Zones way of life, the Mediterranean diet is getting a second turn. Full of whole grains, fruits, vegetables, beans, seeds, nuts, olive oil and fish, this diet is perfectly compared with a Blue Zones lifestyle.

The Mediterranean is instead a general pattern of eating, not just a diet but a way of life which can be narrowed down to two words—whole and simple—because the centerpiece of most dishes are whole, plant-based foods prepared in simple ways.

It has been brought to notice for decades that the Mediterranean Diet offers one of the healthiest eating patterns on earth due to it Olive oil, the abundance of leafy green and the lack of 24- ounces steaks.

The Mediterranean diet (or Med Diet or MD as it's often called) is more than a diet; it's a lifestyle approach to healthy eating. It specifies fruits, vegetables, fish, beans, nuts, and whole grains as well as other ingredients promoting good health such as olive oil and wine.

Types Mediterranean Diet

- Whole grains: this comprises all parts of the grain; the bran, endosperm, and germ. Each of these parts holds healthful nutrients, which disappears when they are refined into products such as white flour; thus, make sure they are as whole grain as possible and don't overdo the amount. Rice, polenta, couscous and quinoa are used a lot in this diet. Pasta, even whole wheat, are requires in small portions. These should be consumed daily and as part of the cornerstone of your meal.

- Vegetables and fruits: often eaten seasonally and locally. This stands to be the largest part and foundation of each meal. Green leafy and colorful vegetables and berries are rich in antioxidants and should be consumed the most. Keep the starchy vegetables to a minimum, such as potatoes, carrots, peas and corn as they are quite high in sugar and lower in fiber. If you are cooking your vegetables, steam or roast them for as short a time as possible. Do not boil them. Fresh fruit is a great satisfying dessert.

- Legumes, nuts, and seeds: serves as the main plant-based source of protein in the diet. Nuts and seeds, such as almonds, pistachios, cashews, walnuts, sunflower, pumpkin and flax seeds, are a delicious and enjoyable snack. Nuts and seeds, however, are high in fat and need to be consumed in reasonable portions.

- Olive oil: this is the main source of fat which replaces less-healthful fats such as butter. Extra Virgin Olive Oil is Use in place of other fats such as butter, margarine and other vegetable oils. If cooking with it, remember that Olive Oil is not recommended for super high heat. It can burn quickly. It is fine for sautéing but don't let it heat too smoking. It is great for roasting vegetables too

- Seafood, poultry, and eggs: these are more consumed more than other meats. Fish has Omega 3 fatty acids, especially fish from wild-caught, cold water sources. Wild fish eat a diet consisting of marine and plant oils that are high in Omega 3. Fish should be consumed at least 2 times weekly. Fish should be baked, grilled or broiled. Do not fry or bread it.

- Dairy: mostly in form of yogurt and cheese, consumed a few times a week. Plain Greek yogurt, feta and goat cheese are great sources of protein, calcium, and good fat sources. Eggs, as fresh as possible, can be consumed 2-3x/week. Milk is restricted in this diet as much as possible. Poultry should be eaten weekly and in small portions. As above, grill, bake or broil your poultry.

- Red wine: consumed moderately with meals. A little red wine is good as long as there are no other reasons you cannot drink alcohol.

- Physical activity: this is done at least 30 minutes a day far the most days of the week.

- Water: taking plenty water regularly helps you to stay hydrated. Water is very important. 6-8 eight-ounce glasses per day.

- Fresh herbs and spices: the type is added to dishes for flavor and color in in place of excess salts.

The following information is from Mediterranean Diet 101: A Meal Plan and Beginner's Guide by Kris Gunnars, BSc – https://authoritynutrition.com/Mediterranean-diet-meal-plan/

Over the years we have seen diets come into enthusiastic favor and then fall dramatically out of favor. It can be extraordinarily frustrating trying to sift through all information and research data that clutters the headlines. As a result, we have forgotten that food and eating should be joyful and simple, not a chore. Mediterranean Diet is the one diet, or style of eating, that consistently come out on top through all the diet mayhem. Studies have shown that people who consume a Mediterranean Diet have lower rates of cardiovascular disease and cancer. This is considered to be due to the emphasis on monounsaturated fats, fruits and vegetables and whole grains. Most significantly, however, people who consume this diet have an easier time managing their weight as the diet is satisfying using real food.

According to research, The Mediterranean Diet scientifically is the traditional diet consumed by people living in the Mediterranean region. This region primarily includes Greece, Italy, Turkey, Spain, southern France, parts of the Middle East and Northern Africa. The diet was founded on foods that were easily cultivated in those regions and other cultural influences. If you travel to those regions today, you will be treated to a fantastic assortment and combination of foods and spices that people have been eating for thousands of years.

The basic premise of the diet is consuming monounsaturated fatty acids, Omega 3 fatty acids, antioxidants, wholegrains, high fiber foods and lots of fruit and vegetables. Balancing the amount of these things is the main tenant of this diet. The study documented the health benefits of a diet "characterized by abundant plant foods (fruit, vegetables, breads, other forms of cereals, potatoes, beans, nuts, and seeds) fresh fruit as the typical daily dessert, olive oil as the principal source of fat, dairy products (principally cheese and yogurt), and fish and poultry consumed in low to moderate amounts, zero to four eggs consumed weekly, red meat consumed in low amounts, and wine consumed in low to moderate amounts, normally with meals. "In subsequent years the body of scientific evidence supporting the healthfulness of the traditional Mediterranean Diet has continued to grow. See all the latest studies at www.oldwayspt.org

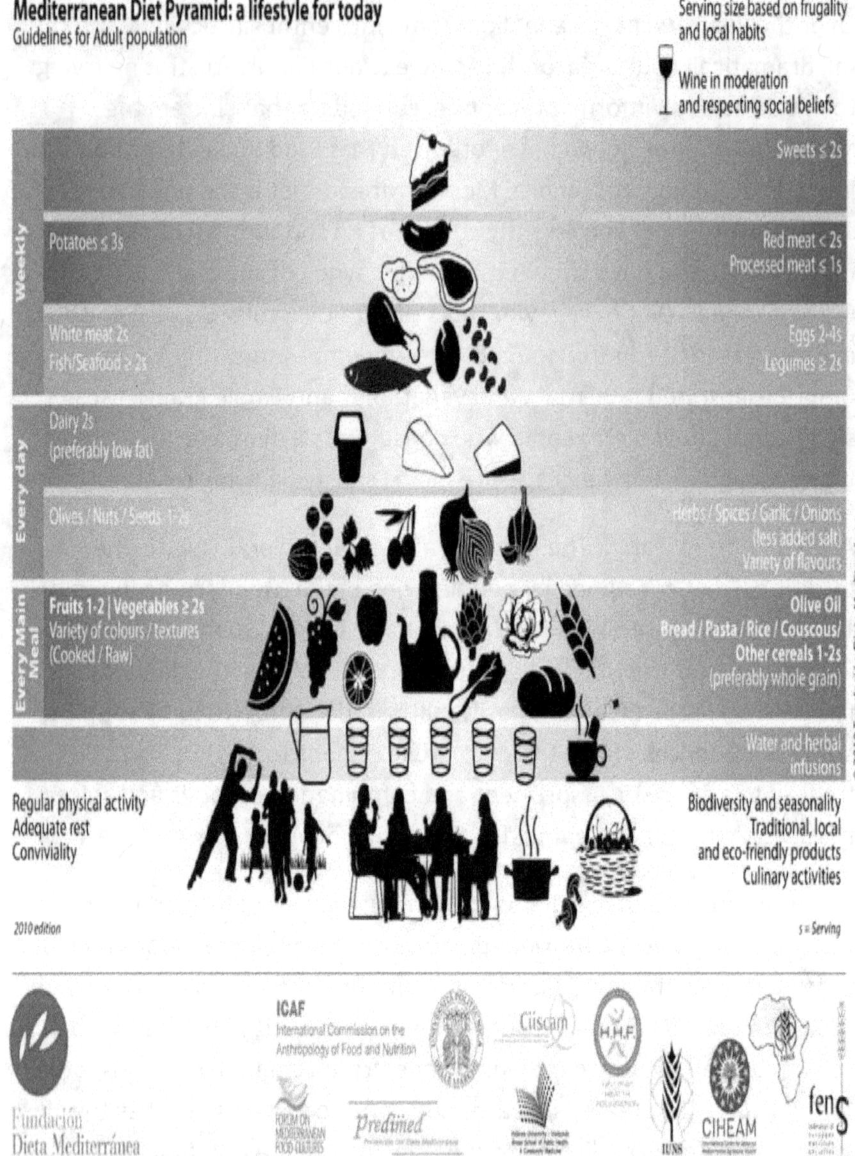

The Mediterranean diet pyramid (source: Fundación Dieta Mediterránea, https://dietamediterranea.com/en/nutrition/)

The Role of the Mediterranean diet in Health and Disease

Research has shown that abundant intake of plant-based foods can be scientifically traced to the prevention of several chronic diseases for example cancers and diabetes, and in turn supply vital nutrients for a wholesome balanced diet. Fruit and vegetables are high in antioxidants and have shown beneficial inflammation reducing effects in the body and brain. More so, antioxidant properties found in some nutrients are considered to be beneficial for protection against neurodegenerative diseases and cardiovascular diseases and in addition to this, it is proposed to presumably help against depression. The largest Mediterranean Diet randomized trial, the Prevención con Dieta Mediterránea (Predimed) trial, in Spain included 7447 men and women, all at high cardiovascular risk at baseline (Estruch et al., 2013). Participants were randomly assigned to either the Mediterranean Diet + extra virgin olive oil group, the Mediterranean Diet + 30g mixed nuts (almonds, hazelnuts, and walnuts) group, or the control group suggested reducing the intake of dietary fat. The trial stopped after nearly 5 years and the two groups assigned to either of the two MediterreanD groups showed large decrease in cardiovascular risk markers such as stroke and myocardial infarction in comparison to the control group. These results are in line with results from the previous Lyon diet heart study which showed that adherence to the Mediterrean Diet reduced the risk of recurrence after a first myocardial infarction. The Mediterrean Diet had a protective effect up to four years after the first infarction. There are indications that risk factors for vascular diseases are also possibly underlying risk factors for cognitive decline, dementia, and AD (Kivipelto et al., 2001; Luchsinger, Noble, & Scarmeas, 2007; Martínez-Lapiscina et al., 2013; Vercambre, Grodstein, Berr, & Kang, 2012). For this reason, the positive effect of the Mediterrean Diet on cardiovascular markers can also be beneficial for vicariously preserving against cognitive decline. Cognitive decline was investigated in relation to the Mediterrean Diet in a cohort of the PREDIMED trial, comprising 522 men and women at high vascular risk. A Spanish validated version of the Mini Mental State Examination (MMSE) (Blesa et al., 2001) and the clock drawing test were utilized to test for neuropsychological aspects (Martínez-Lapiscina et al., 2013). Results showed that participants in the Mediterrean Diet, group + extra virgin olive oil had a higher mean score on the MMSE and the clock drawing test compared to the control group. The MMSE was originally developed by Folstein, Folstein, and Mchugh (1975), adjusted to only measure the cognitive aspect of mental function, hence the "mini". Mood and form of thinking are examples of excluded aspects. The MMSE is divided into two sections, one concerning verbal response and the other regarding the ability to follow verbal and written commands (Folstein et al., 1975). The MMSE is widely used and is high in construct validity (Tombaugh, 1992). In sum, high adherence to the Mediterrean Diet has shown association to decrease total mortality (Trichopoulou, Costacou, Bamia, & Trichopoulos, 2003) and reduced risk of suffering high blood pressure and cardiovascular diseases.

Adherence to the Mediterranean diet and IVF success rate among non-obese women attempting fertility

To begin with, lifestyle factors like diet, smoking, exercise, and stress disrupt reproductive performance. Recent reports have proposed certain preconception dietary habits may influence IVF outcome, such as oocyte and embryo quality, implantation and successful completion of pregnancy.

This book discusses on the role of isolated nutrients or food groups like dairy and whole grains. There are also some epidemiological studies considering nutrition in the light of a more holistic approach that focuses on the role of dietary patterns rather than individual nutrients, foods, or groups, as this approach probably better reflects long-term eating habits and behaviors. Among dietary patterns, the Mediterranean diet (MD), a diet rich in vegetables, fruits, whole grains, legumes, nuts and olive oil, and low in red meat, seems encouraging and at all account recognize for its positive effects on human health. Previously, investigation the association between preconception dietary patterns and IVF outcomes among sub fertile couples in the Netherlands, has shown that high adherence by the couple to a 'Mediterranean' type pattern (defined using principal component analysis) increased the probability of pregnancy. A comparable effect for the adherence to a healthy diet and the chance of ongoing pregnancy following IVF was subsequently found in a Dutch cohort of couples receiving their first IVF treatment, by calculating a preconception dietary risk score based on dietary recommendations of the Netherlands Nutrition Centre (Twigt et al.,

2012). Never the less, adequate studies may be required to verify the beneficial role of a Mediterrean Diet on assisted reproductive performance in other populations. Moreover, obesity's has high impact on female reproductive potential, it is extremely vital to make clear the role and the potential mechanism(s) by which Mediterrean Diet specifically may wield beneficial effects on assisted reproduction outcome beyond body weight.

Hence, the present study explores potential associations between Mediterrean Diet and IVF clinical outcomes among non-obese women of infertile couples attempting fertility. We hypothesized that greater adherence to the Mediterrean Diet, which was defined using an a-priori dietary pattern approach and calculation of the validated Mediterranean diet score according to (MedDietScore)...
http://academic.oup.com/humrep

Non-Communicable Disease (NCD)

The leading cause of death globally is Non-Communicable Disease; this is responsible for 68% of the total deaths and 16 million premature deaths (i.e. those occurring before the age of 70 years) each year according to (Non communicable diseases progress monitor. Geneva: World Health Organization; 2015).

 The four main types of Non communicable disease include cancer, cardiovascular diseases (CVD; including heart attack and stroke), chronic respiratory disease (e.g. asthma, chronic obstructive pulmonary disease) and diabetes. Deaths rate from NCDs is originally envisaged to increase from 38 million worldwide in 2012 to 52 million by 2030. Following the first High-level Meeting of the General Assembly on the Prevention and Control of Non communicable Diseases in 2011, governments declared a commitment to reducing NCD risk factors and creating health-promoting environments by introducing policies and actions aimed at promoting healthy diets. In 2013, WHO produced a NCD Global Monitoring Framework that included nine global targets for 2025 (against a 2010 baseline), of which target 7 is to "halt the rise in diabetes and obesity". The 2030 Agenda for Sustainable Development also recognizes the global impact of NCDs, setting a target to reduce premature deaths from NCDs by one third by 2030 (Sustainable Development Goal (SDG) target 3.4). Of the six WHO regions, the WHO European Region is the one most affected by NCDs. The prevalence and associated mortality for NCDs are high across all 53 Member States of the WHO European Region for which data are available, despite differences in their economic, social and political conditions. The four main types of NCDs account for an estimated 86% of deaths and 77% of disease burden in this Region. In 2012, Health 2020 was adopted by all Member States of the Region with the aim to "significantly improve the health and well-being of populations, reduce health inequalities, strengthen public health, and ensure people-centered health systems that are universal, equitable, sustainable, and of high quality". Inspired by the Health 2020 vision, the European Food and Nutrition Action Plan 2015–2020 focuses on reducing preventable diet-related NCDs and all other forms of malnutrition prevalent in the Region. It calls for a whole-of-government, health-in-all-policies approach, and it outlines a set of priority actions that contribute to improved food system governance, and population diet and nutritional status.

The key objectives of the European Food and Nutrition Action Plan 2015–2020 (European food and nutrition action plan 2015–2020. Copenhagen; WHO Regional Office for Europe; 2014 (EUR/RC64/R7)) are to:

- create healthy food and drink environments.

- promote the gains of a healthy diet throughout the life-course, especially for the most vulnerable groups;

- reinforce health systems to promote healthy diets;

- support surveillance, monitoring, evaluation and research; and

- strengthen governance, intersectoral alliances and networks for a health-in all-policies approach.

Together, these initiatives have created positive momentum for reducing Non communicable Diseases in the lead-up to the third High-level Meeting of the General Assembly on Non communicable Diseases in 2018.

Despite the overwhelming and increasing burden of Non communicable Diseases or NCD, a mere 1% of global health financing is directed towards Non communicable Diseases related programs. This trend is reflected in the Region, with most Member States allocating limited funds for Non communicable Disease prevention and health promotion activities. More encouragingly, however, 97% of health ministries have a Non communicable Disease prevention and control unit or department. Investment in Non communicable Disease prevention is important because 80% of premature heart disease, stroke and type 2 diabetes cases is preventable.

The biggest killers in the Region, cancer and CVD, are both influenced by unhealthy diets. The leading risk factors for diet-related NCDs are excess consumption of unhealthy fats, sugar and salt and low consumption of fresh fruit and vegetables. These NCDs accounted for 27% of all deaths in the Region in 2015. National surveys in most European countries indicate excessive fat intake, low fruit, and vegetable intake, and increasing rates of overweight and obesity. In 2011, governments made a commitment to reducing NCD risk factors, creating health-promoting environments and strengthening national policies in the Political Declaration of the High-level Meeting of the General Assembly on the Prevention and Control of Noncommunicable Diseases. Health-promoting activities based on diet and nutrition are now widespread throughout the Region. The recent release of the European Food and Nutrition Action Plan 2015–2020 , the announcement of the United Nations Decade of Action on Nutrition and the subsequent increase in global attention may further increase the volume, capacity and funds for these and related activities to effectively tackle diet-related NCDs.

NCD rates are rising in low- and high-income countries alike. No country has reduced obesity rates in the past 33 years. This poses a significant economic burden: CVD costs European Union countries €169 billion; cancer costs €124 billion annually; and obesity accounts for 2–8% of overall health costs. Moreover, global issues such as climate change, conflict, migration and political instability threaten to exacerbate NCD morbidity and mortality rates. Obesity and type 2 diabetes. Obesity rates are high or increasing worldwide and no country is on track to achieve voluntary target 7 of the NCD Global Monitoring Framework ; Iceland and Malta are the only two European countries on course to halt the rise in type 2 diabetes; and Liechtenstein, Monaco and San Marino have no data available on overweight, obesity and type 2 diabetes .

Conflict and migration. The risks associated with population movement from regions of conflict both predispose individuals to developing NCDs and worsen pre-existing chronic conditions. The associated psychological stress, reproductive health issues, drug and alcohol abuse, interruption of health services, food insecurity and nutrition disorders all increase NCD vulnerability.

Climate change. Climate change poses a catastrophic risk to human health by exacerbating the global burden of NCDs. Of note is the threat that climate change poses to healthy food systems. Unpredictable and unfavorable weather patterns threaten food security, most notably the availability and cost of health-promoting fresh fruits and vegetables.

Political instability. A unified, whole-of-government approach to NCD prevention is the best way to ensure sustained and stable funding, resources and public health and research priorities. Therefore, political instability can threaten efforts to reduce the NCD burden.

Population ageing. Populations are ageing rapidly worldwide but increased longevity is not always accompanied by good health. Although older people contribute to society in many ways, an ageing population increases the burden on health care systems. For example, it is estimated that over 75 million people will be living with dementia in 2030, and this figure expected to triple by 2050 (World report on ageing and health. Geneva: World Health Organization; 2015).

The beneficial effects of Mediterranean Diet against Non Communicable Disease

It is undoubtably confirmed that unhealthy diet is the principal predominant cause of ill health globally and a significant variable risk factor for NCDs, especially cancer, CVD, and type 2 diabetes. The health-promoting properties of Mediterranean Diets has been studied extensively: the popularity of the MD is one without compare, attracting consciously the attention of the general population and the universal media.

The origin of MD can be traced back to the olive-growing areas of the Mediterranean region with strong cultural association with these areas. Various definitions have developed as the MD has been adopted beyond the Mediterranean region and become increasingly medicalized as both a treatment and a prevention intervention. Despite these variations, the MD remains based on fresh, seasonal and local food. Correspondently with the MD pyramid above, the diet is characterized by a high intake of plant-based foods (fruit, vegetables, nuts and cereals) and olive oil; a moderate intake of fish and poultry; a low intake of dairy products (principally yoghurt and cheese), red meat, processed meats and sweets (for which fresh fruit is often substituted); and a moderate wine intake, normally consumed with meals.

Social and cultural factors closely associated with the traditional MD, including shared eating practices, post-meal siestas (afternoon naps) and lengthy mealtimes, are also thought to contribute to the attributed positive health effects recorded in the Mediterranean region. The recommendation to practice conviviality (i.e. the quality of being friendly and lively) continues to form part of the modern-day MD pyramid. In 2010, the MD in Croatia, Cyprus, Greece, Italy, Morocco, Portugal, and Spain was inscribed on the United Nations Educational, Scientific and Cultural Organization's Representative List of the Intangible Cultural Heritage of Humanity.

The MD is inversely associated with all-cause mortality and has been associated to numerous health benefits, including a lower incidence of cancer, cognitive disease, and CVD, as well as for metabolic syndrome, obesity, and type 2 diabetes. Despite abundant literature in this field, the most widely researched health benefits of the MD relate to CVD, reflecting the high global burden. Research suggests that the following NCDs and intermediate risk factors can be reduced, prevented or treated by the MD. Thus;

- **Cancer.** Strict adherence to the MD is significantly associated with a lower risk of all-cause cancer mortality, specifically breast, colorectal, gastric, head and neck, and prostate cancer. Reinforcing the importance of dietary factors in gastric carcinogenesis, the European Prospective Investigation into

Cancer and Nutrition (EPIC) study has demonstrated a strong association between MD adherence and reduced cancer risk.

- **Cognitive disease**. Strict adherence to the MD is associated with a reduced risk of developing Alzheimer's and Parkinson's diseases and is reported to slow or halt the progression of a range of cognitive diseases from mild cognitive impairment to Alzheimer's disease.
- **Cardiovascular Disease**. The Prevención con Dieta Mediterránea (PREDIMED; Prevention with the Mediterranean Diet) study investigated the effects of the MD in the primary prevention of CVD (43). It found that a MD containing nuts reduced the mortality risk of CVD, myocardial infarction and stroke by 30%; the MD containing olive oil reduced CVD by 30%; and the risk of stroke was reduced by 49% compared with a reference group on a low-fat diet based on American Heart Association guidelines. PREDIMED and other studies support the benefits of the MD in the primary prevention of CVD. The beneficial effects of the MD on cardiovascular health are transferable to non-Mediterranean populations.
- **Type 2 diabetes**. The benefits of the MD on type 2 diabetes are twofold: prevention in unaffected individuals and improved glycemic control in patients with established diabetes. Studies have demonstrated that MD intervention is associated with a 52% reduction in diabetes incidence in patients with high-risk CVD, a delayed requirement for drug therapy in newly diagnosed overweight patients and improved blood glucose levels. Compared with low-fat diets based on American Heart Association guidelines, the MD appears to be more beneficial for patients with type 2 diabetes.

The publication strongly suggests that Mediterranean-like dietary patterns are extremely commendable in preventing and controlling diet-related NCDs, there by presenting a strong point for their high adoption.

Impact of Mediterrean Diet

Research into the impact of MD policies on NCDs were found for only three countries: Norway, Spain, and Sweden. This review assessed the impact of national MD based guidelines, recommendations or pyramids on NCDs. Together, they provide examples of adaptable tools and methods for assessing the health impact of MD based dietary guidelines. Spanish dietary guidelines Spain's food pyramid and dietary recommendations promote the traditional MD through three key messages:

(i) Eat good fats found in foods such as fish, nuts and olive oil.
(ii) Eat plenty of cereals in preference to whole grain.
(iii) Finally try to eat five portions of fruits and vegetables every day.

Using the 2004 revised version of the Spanish food pyramid score to measure guideline adherence of questionnaire results.

Molina-Montes et al. concluded that the guidelines might act as an effective obesity prevention tool in countries with rising rates of obesity. Increased adherence was associated with lower odds of obesity (body mass index: >30 kg/m2) and abdominal adiposity (waist circumference: >102 cm for men, >88 cm for women), which are key risk factors for CVD, diabetes and some cancers. 2.2.2. Swedish dietary guidelines. The Swedish national dietary guidelines are based on the 2012 NNR, with consideration of Swedish food culture and the ability of local consumers to adhere to recommendations.

The guidelines promote three key messages:

(i) Eat more berries, fish, fruit, nuts, seeds, shellfish and vegetables.
(ii) Switch to whole grains, healthy fats (i.e. rapeseed oil) and low-fat dairy products.
(iii) And eat less red and processed meat, as well as less salt, sugar, and alcohol.

In accordance, the study found that adherence to the high-quality diet may reduce the risk of CVD events (by 32% in men and 27% in women).

Effect of Mediterrean Diet on life span

 In relation to numerous studies, it has been revealed that the Mediterranean Diet helps prevent heart disease and cancer. At some point in the 1960's many Mediterranean countries had the highest life expectancies in the world. Today the Italian island of Sardinia and the Greek island of Ikaria are two of the five identified blue zones in the world. A blue zone is a location in which its inhabitants live much longer lives. This may be attributed to genes but also to the Mediterranean diet and lifestyle: plant based diet, physical activity and plenty of social contact.

The diet includes certain "ingredients" that have been associated consistently with longevity, better heart and cognitive health. The "longevity ingredients" in this eating pattern are vegetables, plants in the form of greens and herbs, legumes, fish, dairy from free-range animals, olive oil as the main source of fat, very little meat and a bit of alcohol.

Inclusively, several studies have been associated with Mediterranean diet promoting longevity. Few years back, a comprehensive literature review conducted by Italian researchers on an overall population of over 4,000,000 showed that a Mediterranean diet can reduce risk of death by 8%. The EPIC Elderly Study which included information of over 74,000 Europeans showed that adherence to a Mediterranean diet was associated with lower mortality. Another study that analyzed and compared the diets of centenarians from the Sicani Mountains in Sicily who had a close adherence to the Mediterranean diet with those of Palermo residents who were following a more westernized diet, found that adherence to the diet had a significant effect on mortality. It was noted that low animal protein, low glycemic index and high polyphenol content regulates and influences certain pathways and chemicals of the body that are involved in longevity.

More so, longevity is not only associated with Mediterranean populations, but also inhabitants of other countries who follow a Mediterranean diet. A large study that involved over 400,000 men and women in the United States, found that high adherence to a Mediterranean style diet reduced the risk of death from all cause including cardiovascular disease and cancer. In another study, Swedish researchers investigated the relationship of the Mediterranean diet with mortality in a Swedish population and found that the diet also had a positive effect on the Swedish as well, increasing longevity. In yet another study in Switzerland, it was also found that following a Mediterranean diet was associated with lower mortality. In other words the benefits of longevity associated with a Mediterranean diet can be experienced anywhere in the world.

A recent study from the Brigham and Women's Hospital, a teaching hospital of Harvard Medical School, provides additional evidence that this eating style promotes longevity. Published in the British Medical Journal, the study included data from 4,676 women from the Nurses' Health Study – an ongoing study running since 1976 that has been following over 120,000 nurses from the United States. They found that those who followed a Mediterranean style diet had longer telomeres. Telomeres are found at the ends of chromosomes and protect from deterioration. Longer telomeres have been associated with longer life.

It is extremely important to take in consideration that when we talk of the Mediterranean diet and longevity, we are not only referring to an actual diet, but to a lifestyle. The high life expectancy observed in these areas and populations, is associated with the lifestyle. This includes social networks, eating together, taking naps, less urgency and of course physical activity. While replicating a Mediterranean lifestyle may seem unrealistic, there are several components one can adopt, even with today's busy schedule. Strategies on how to incorporate the Mediterranean diet and lifestyle for a US population will be discussed at the Mediterranean Diet Roundtable.

The Mediterranean diet represents the gold Standard in preventive medicine, probably due to the harmonic combination of many elements with antioxidant and anti-inflammatory properties, which overwhelm any single nutrient or food item. The whole seems more important than the sum of its parts

A Mediterranean diet with either olive oil or nuts may reduce the combined risk of stroke, heart attack, and death from heart disease.

However, research shows that the incidence of heart disease seems to be lower among people living in Italy, Greece, and other countries around the Mediterranean, compared with those living in the United States. Studies suggest that diet may play a role. People around the Mediterranean have traditionally followed a diet that's rich in plant-based foods, including fruits, vegetables, whole grains, breads, legumes, potatoes, nuts, and seeds. The main dietary fat is extra virgin olive oil, and people also consume moderate amounts of red wine, fish, poultry, dairy, and eggs. Meanwhile, red meat plays only a small part. This eating pattern has started to become popular around the world as a means to improve health and prevent disease.

we should eat foods that leave us energized, reduce our risk of illness, and allow us to maintain a healthy weight. To live longer and be healthier, we have to fuel our bodies with nutrient-dense foods. Natural plant foods can restore our health and vitality.

Ten best food for longevity

1. Cruciferous Vegetables

These are vegetable powerhouses with the unique ability to modify human hormones, activate the body's natural detoxification system and inhibit the growth of cancerous cells. Cruciferous vegetables should be chewed thoroughly or eaten shredded, chopped, juiced or blended in order to release their potent anti-cancer properties. The cruciferous phytochemical sulforaphane has been found to protect blood vessel walls from inflammatory signaling that can lead to heart disease. Cruciferous vegetables are the most nutrient-dense of all the foods. Eat a variety in both raw and cooked form daily — try some broccoli, cauliflower, Brussels sprouts, kale or cabbage.

2. Salad Greens

These includes raw, leafy green vegetables – some are cruciferous – contain less than 100 calories per pound, making them an ideal food for weight control. In scientific studies, women who ate a large salad at the beginning of a meal ate fewer calories from the rest of the meal, and larger salads reduced calories more than smaller ones. In addition to keeping weight down, greater intake of salads, leafy greens or raw vegetables is associated with reduced risk of heart attack, stroke, diabetes and several cancers. Leafy greens are also rich in the essential B-vitamin folate plus lutein and zeaxanthin, carotenoids that protect the eyes from light damage. Try kale, collard greens, mustard greens, spinach or lettuce. To maximize the health benefits of leafy greens, you must maximize your absorption of their fat-soluble phytochemicals, carotenoids in particular, and that requires fats – which is why your salad (or dressing) should always contain nuts and/or seeds.

3. **Nuts**

A high-nutrient source of healthful fats, plant protein, fiber, antioxidants, phytosterols and minerals, nuts are a low-glycemic food that also help reduce the glycemic load of an entire meal, making them an important component for an anti-diabetes diet. Despite their caloric density, nut consumption is associated with lower body weight, potentially due to appetite suppression from heart-healthy components. Eating nuts regularly also reduces cholesterol and is linked to a 35 percent reduction in the risk of heart disease. Top your next salad with chopped walnuts or sliced almonds or blend some raw cashews into a creamy salad dressing.

4. **Seeds**

The nutritional profile of seeds is very similar to nuts in that they provide healthy fats, minerals and antioxidants, but seeds have more protein and are abundant in trace minerals. Flax, chia and hemp seeds are rich in omega-3 fats. Flax, chia and sesame seeds are also rich lignans, breast cancer-fighting phytoestrogens. Sesame seeds are rich in calcium and vitamin E and pumpkin seeds are especially rich in zinc. For maximum nutritional benefits, nuts and seeds should be eaten raw or only lightly toasted. Try adding flax or chia seeds to your morning smoothie or oatmeal.

5. Berries

These antioxidant-rich fruits are very heart-healthy. Studies in which participants ate blueberries or strawberries daily for several weeks reported improvements in blood pressure, signs of oxidative stress, total and LDL cholesterol. Berries also have anti-cancer properties and are an excellent food for the brain. There is evidence that berry consumption could help prevent cognitive decline with aging. Stick with the tried and traditional strawberry or blueberry, or try something new like goji berries.

6. Pomegranate

The pomegranate is a unique fruit, containing tiny, crisp, juicy arils with a tasty mix of sweet and tart flavors. The signature phytochemical of pomegranate, punicalagin, is the most abundant and is responsible for more than half the antioxidant activity of pomegranate juice. Pomegranate phytochemicals have a variety of anti-cancer, cardio-protective and brain-healthy actions. Most notably, a study of patients with severe carotid artery blockages who drank one ounce of pomegranate juice daily for one year found a 30 percent reduction in atherosclerotic plaque; in the control group, atherosclerotic plaque increased by nine percent. In another study of older adults, those who drank pomegranate juice daily for 28 days performed better on a memory task compared to those who drank a placebo beverage. Tip: To remove the edible arils from the fruit, score it around a half inch deep on the diameter, twist to split it in two and pound the back with the back of a large spoon.

7. Beans

Daily consumption of beans and other legumes helps stabilize blood sugar, reduce your appetite and protect against colon cancer. The most nutrient-dense starch source, beans act as an anti-diabetes and weight-loss food because they are digested slowly, which blunts the rise in blood glucose after a meal and helps prevent food cravings by promoting satiety. They also contain lots of soluble fiber which helps lower cholesterol, and resistant starch which is converted by intestinal bacteria into short-chain fatty acids that help prevent colon cancer. Eating beans, peas or lentils twice a week has been found to decrease colon cancer risk by 50 percent. Legume consumption also provides significant protection against other cancers too. Red beans, black beans, chickpeas, lentils, split peas – they are all good, so sample them all and decide on your own favorites.

8. Mushrooms

Consuming mushrooms regularly is associated with a decreased risk of breast cancer. Because they contain aromatase inhibitors, compounds that inhibit the production of estrogen, white and portobello mushrooms are especially protective against breast cancer. Mushrooms have quite an array of beneficial properties. Studies on different types of mushrooms have found anti-inflammatory effects, enhanced immune cell activity, prevention of DNA damage, slowed cancer cell growth and angiogenesis inhibition. Mushrooms should always be cooked; raw mushrooms contain a potentially carcinogenic substance called agaritine that is significantly reduced by cooking. Regularly include common white mushrooms in your diet and try some of the more exotic varieties like shiitake, oyster, maitake or reishi.

9. Onions and Garlic

The allium family of vegetables, of which onions are a member, benefit the cardiovascular and immune systems and have anti-diabetic and anti-cancer effects. Increased consumption of allium vegetables is associated with a lower risk of gastric and prostate cancers. These vegetables are known for their organosulfur compounds which help prevent the development of cancers by detoxifying carcinogens, halting cancer cell growth and blocking angiogenesis. These compounds are released when they are chopped, crushed or chewed. Onions also contain high concentrations of health-promoting flavonoid antioxidants, which have anti-inflammatory effects that may contribute to cancer prevention. In addition to garlic and yellow onions, try leeks, chives, shallots and scallions.

10. Tomatoes

An abundance of health-promoting nutrients can be found in tomatoes – lycopene, vitamins C and E, beta-carotene and flavanol antioxidants, to name but a few. Lycopene in particular protects against prostate cancer, UV skin damage and cardiovascular disease. About 85 percent of the lycopene in American diets is derived from tomatoes. Lycopene is more absorbable when tomatoes are cooked – one cup of tomato sauce has 10 times the lycopene as one cup of raw, chopped tomatoes. Also keep in mind that carotenoids, like lycopene, are best absorbed when accompanied by healthy fats, so enjoy your tomatoes in a salad with nuts or a nut-based dressing for extra nutritional punch. Tip: buy diced and crushed tomatoes in glass jars, not cans, to avoid the endocrine disruptor BPA in can liners

The Blue Zone Diet

Dan Buettner, Founder of Blue Zones said "I have traveled the world for National Geographic to identify the diet, eating patterns, and lifestyles of the world's longest-lived people. The Blue Zones Meal Planner makes it easy for everyone to eat in a way that gives them the best chance to live to 100." He added. In wide geographical definition, Blue Zone can be defined as an area where people are either reaching age 100 at extraordinary rates, have the highest life expectancy, or the lowest rate of middle age mortality. One might wonder how they were able to achieve this; Blue Zone diet. Blue Zone diets are primarily plant – based, with as much as 95% of daily food intake coming from vegetables, fruits, grains, and legumes. As such people in Blue Zone avoid meat and dairy, as well as sugary foods and beverages and they also steer clear of processed foods.

Blue Zone Diet further envisage exercise with nature walks in the forest to take in pine tree nutrients. They are religious group in Linda Vista. Others that follow similar calm and health diet live in Japan and others South America. Eating organic foods, low stress lives, and inner peace and prayers.

Blue zone diet is very intriguing because of the quality of life and the longevity of the people living life style diet. Being time poor is no excuse.

The Blue Zone diet should give the average person 10 extra years of life expectancy –that's about 90000 hours over the course of your life

This principle identifies common themes in the diets of those living in the Blue Zones – areas throughout the world with a higher ratio of centenarians. This area is mainly plant based but some areas have more seafood. Blue Zones centenarians tend to eat meat dishes – usually pork or chicken – only once a week or even less, with meat often considered a celebratory meal. Midday meal is the main one of the days, the evening meal is considered the smallest. Bear I mind that Blue zone diet is considered more than food – it's undeniably a way of life. Take into account that there is no one right way to eat affordable and sustainable. People in the Blue Zones often saved meat meals for celebrations and were mainly, but not exclusively, vegetarians. "Blue Zoners weren't absolutists. We know that eating a lot of meat – say two servings a day or more – may triple your chances of diabetes, cancer, or heart disease, but eating very little – fewer than five times a month – probably won't hurt you. "Creating an environment that makes it easier to eat more plants might be something as basic as making a new vegetarian friend.

10 Blue Zones Food Guidelines

Accepting and practicing some of the healthy eating principles into your routine, will improve and promote your health for longevity. Guidelines for consumption of in Blue Zone includes:

- 95/5 RULE Eat Plants. 95 percent of your food should be fruits, vegetables, grains, greens, beans, and fruits. Use olive oil to sauté and spices flavor vegetables. Feel free to eat a cup (cooked) of whole grains daily.

- LIMIT MEAT Think of meat as a celebratory food. Portions should be no larger than a deck of cards, once or twice a week. Avoid processed meats such as hot dogs, bacon and sausages.

- FISH IS FINE Enjoy fish up to three times weekly. Wild-caught salmon or smaller fish like sardines, trout, snapper, cod, and anchovies are okay choices. Limit portion sizes to 3 ounces (about the size of the palm of your hand.)

- DIMINISH DAIRY Avoid dairy when possible. If cheese is a must, try ice-cube size portions of sheep (pecorino) or goat (feta) cheese to flavor foods. If you eat eggs, limit intake to 3/week.

- DAILY DOSE OF BEANS Eat a cup of beans daily spread out across breakfast, lunch or dinner. All beans count, including tofu. They contain high quality protein and fiber. If you buy canned beans, avoid added salt, sugar and chemicals.

- SLASH SUGAR Consume only 28 grams (7 teaspoons) of added sugar daily. Reserve cookies, cakes, and candies for special occasions. Read labels and avoid foods with more than 8 grams of sugar. Make honey your go-to sweetener.

- SNACK ON NUTS Eat a handful of nuts daily: almonds, pistachios, walnuts, hazelnuts, sunflower seeds, pumpkin seeds, Brazil nuts, and peanuts. Try different nuts so you don't tire of them. Avoid sugar-coated nuts.

- SOUR ON BREAD Eat only 100% whole grain breads or authentic sourdough bread made from live cultures. Limit bread to two slices daily. Chose whole grain corn tortillas over flour tortillas. Avoid white breads and wraps.

- GO WHOLLY WHOLE Try to eat only whole foods or processed foods with fewer than 5 ingredients: If it's manufactured in a plant, avoid it. If it comes from a plant, eat it.

- DRINK MOSTLY WATER Drink six glasses of water daily. Feel free to drink unsweetened teas and coffee. Enjoy Wine at 5 with friends or with Blue Zones inspired meals. Avoid all sugar-sweetened and diet sodas.

Guidelines to adherence to Blue Zone Diet

Guidelines to crowd out refined starches and sugar, replacing them with more wholesome, nutrient- dense, and fiber.

Plant Slant

It is important to endeavor that 95% of your food comes from a plant or a plant product.

Limit animal protein in your diet to no more than one small serving per day. Adhering to the intake of plant product example favor beans, greens, yams and sweet potatoes, fruits, nuts, and seeds. Whole grains are okay too. While people in four of the five Blue Zones consume meat, they do so sparingly, using it as a celebratory food, a small side, or a way to flavor dishes. Walter Willett of the Harvard School of Public Health concluded by saying: "Meat is like radiation: We don't know the safe level." Undoubtedly, research suggests that 30-year-old vegetarian Adventists will likely outlive their meat-eating counterparts by as many as eight years. At the same time, adequate amount of plant-based foods in your meals has many beneficial health effects. In the blue zones people eat an impressive variety of garden vegetables when they are in season, and then they pickle or dry the surplus to enjoy during the off-season. The best of the best longevity foods in the Blue Zones diet are leafy greens such as spinach, kale, beet and turnip tops, chard, and collards. In Ikaria more than 75 varieties of edible greens grow like weeds; many contain ten times the polyphenols found in red wine. Studies have found that middle-aged people who consumed the equivalent of a cup of cooked greens daily were half as likely to die in the next four years as those who ate no greens. It is of opinion that people who consumed a quarter pound of fruit daily (about an apple) were 60% less likely to die during the next four years than those who didn't, this was discovered by some researchers. Many oils derive from plants, and they are all preferable to animal-based fats. We cannot say that olive oil is the only healthy plant-based oil, but it is the one most often used in the Blue Zones diet. Evidence shows that olive oil consumption increases good cholesterol and lowers bad cholesterol.

Protein in the Blue Zones Diet

It has already been established that our bodies need protein for strong bones and muscle development—but the right amount is not clear. The average American woman consumes 70 grams of protein daily, the average man more than 100 grams, which is absolutely too much. The Centers for Disease Control and Prevention recommends 46 to 56 grams per day. But quantity is of no importance but quality. We also need the right kind of protein. Protein—also known as amino acids—comes in 21 varieties. Of those, the body can't make nine, which are called the nine "essential" amino acids because we need them and must get them from our diet. Meat and eggs will provide all nine amino acids, while few plant food sources do. But meat and eggs also deliver fat and cholesterol, which tend to promote heart disease and cancer. For this reason to eat the Blue Zones diet and emphasize plant-based foods, indeed "pairing" certain foods together is the trick .Combination of the right plant foods, will definitely obtain all the essential amino acids. Not only does this meet your protein needs but also keep your calorie intake in check.

Retreat from Meat

Meat consumption should be limited to at most twice a week. Eat meat twice a week or even less in servings sized no more than two ounces cooked. Favor true free-range chicken and family-farmed pork or lamb instead of meats raised industrially. Avoid processed meats like hot dogs, luncheon meats, or sausages. In most Blue Zones diets people ate small amounts of pork, chicken, or lamb. (Adventists, the one exception, ate no meat at all.) Families traditionally slaughtered their pig or goat for festival celebrations, ate heartily, and preserved the leftovers, which they would then use sparingly as fat for frying or as a condiment for flavor. Chickens roamed on the land, eating grubs and roosting freely. But chicken meat, likewise, was a rare treat savored over many meals. Averaging out meat consumption over all Blue Zones, we found that people were eating small amounts of meat, about two ounces or less at a time, about five times per month. About once a month they splurged, usually on roasted pig or goat. Neither beef nor turkey figures significantly into the average Blue Zones diet.

Free-Range Meats

The meat people in the blue zones eat comes from free-roaming animals. These animals are not dosed with hormones, pesticides, or antibiotics and do not experience the misery of big feedlots. Goats graze continually on grasses, foliage, and herbs. Sardinian and Ikarian pigs eat kitchen scraps and forage for wild acorns and roots. These traditional husbandry practices likely produce meat with higher levels of healthy omega-3 fatty acids than the rich meat of grain-fed animals.

On the on other hand, it is not certain if people lived longer because they ate a little bit of meat as part of the Blue Zones diet or if they thrived despite it. There are so many healthy practices blue zones people engaged in, they may have been able to get away with a little meat now and then because its deleterious effect was counterbalanced by other food and lifestyle choices.

Fish Is Fine

Intake of three ounces of fish daily is certainly a good idea .Think of three ounces as about the size of a deck of cards before it is cooked. It is important to select fish that are common and abundant, not threatened by overfishing. The Adventist Health Study 2, which has been following 96,000 Americans since 2002, found that the people who lived the longest were not vegans or meat-eaters. They were "pesco-vegetarians," or pescatarians, people who ate a plant-based diet including a small portion of fish, up to once daily. In other Blue Zones diets, fish was a common part of everyday meals, eaten on average two to three times a week. There are other ethical and health considerations involved in including fish in your diet. In the world's blue zones, in most cases, the fish being eaten are small, relatively inexpensive fish such as sardines, anchovies, and cod—middle-of-the-food-chain species that are not exposed to the high levels of mercury or other chemicals like PCBs that pollute our gourmet fish supply today. People in the blue zones don't overfish the waters as corporate fisheries do, threatening to deplete entire species. Blue zones fishermen cannot afford to wreak havoc on the ecosystems they depend on. There is no Blue Zones diet evidence favoring any particular fish, though, including salmon.

Diminish Dairy

Minimize your consumption of cow's milk and dairy products such as cheese, cream, and butter. In terms of the human diet, dairy is a relative newcomer, introduced about 8,000 to 10,000 years ago. Our digestive systems are not optimized for milk or milk products (other than human milk), and now we recognize that the number of people who (often unknowingly) have some difficulty digesting lactose may be as high as 60%. Arguments against milk often focus on its high fat and sugar content. Neal Barnard, the founder and president of the Physicians Committee for Responsible Medicine, points out that 49% of the calories in whole milk and about 70% of the calories in cheese come from fat—and that much of this fat is saturated. All milk has lactose sugar as well. About 55% of the calories in skim milk come from lactose sugar, for example. While Americans have relied on milk for calcium and protein for decades, in the Blue Zones diet people get these nutrients from plant-based sources. One cup of cooked kale or two-thirds of a cup of tofu, for instance, provides just as much bioavailable calcium as a cup of milk. Small amounts of sheep's milk or goat's milk products—especially full-fat, naturally fermented yogurt with no added sugars—a few times weekly are okay in a Blue Zones diet. Goat's and sheep's milk products do figure prominently in the traditional menus of both the Ikarian and Sardinian Blue Zones. We don't know if it's the goat's milk or sheep's milk that makes people healthier or if it's the fact that people in the blue zones climb up and down the same hilly terrain as the goats. Interestingly, most goat's milk in the Blue Zones diet is consumed not as liquid but as fermented products such as yogurt, sour milk, or cheese. Although goat's milk contains lactose, it also contains lactase, an enzyme that helps the body digest lactose.

Occasional Egg

Limit egg consumption to no more than three eggs per week. Eggs are consumed in all five Blue Zones diets, where people eat them an average of two to four times per week. As with meat protein, the egg is a side dish, eaten alongside a larger portion of a whole-grain or other plant-based feature. Nicoyans fry an egg to fold into a corn tortilla with a side of beans. Okinawans boil an egg in their soup. People in the Mediterranean blue zones fry an egg as a side dish with bread, almonds, and olives for breakfast. Eggs in the Blue Zones diet come from chickens that range freely, eat a wide variety of natural foods, do not receive hormones or antibiotics, and produce slowly matured eggs that are naturally higher in omega-3 fatty acids. Factory-produced eggs come to maturity about twice as fast as eggs laid by breeds of chickens in the blue zones. Eggs provide a complete protein that includes amino acids necessary for your body plus B vitamins, vitamins A, D, and E, and minerals such as selenium. Data from the Adventist Health Study 2 showed that egg-eating vegetarians lived slightly longer than vegans (though they tended to weigh more). There are other health concerns that might influence your decision to eat eggs as part of your Blue Zones diet. Diabetics need to be cautious about consuming egg yolks, and egg consumption has been correlated to higher rates of prostate cancer for men and exacerbated kidney problems for women. There is still a debate about the effect of dietary cholesterol on arteries, but some people with heart or circulatory problems waive them despite expert argument.

Daily Dose of Beans

Endeavour to consume at least a half cup of cooked beans daily. Beans are the cornerstone of every Blue Zones diet in the world: black beans in Nicoya; lentils, garbanzo, and white beans in the Mediterranean; and soybeans in Okinawa. The long-lived populations in these blue zones eat at least four times as many beans as we do, on average. One five-country study, financed by the World Health Organization, found that eating 20 grams of beans daily reduced a person's risk of dying in any given year by about 8%. The fact is beans represent the consummate superfood in the Blue Zones diet. On average, they are made up of 21% protein, 77% complex carbohydrates (the kind that deliver a slow and steady energy, rather than the spike you get from refined carbohydrates like white flour), and only a few percent fat. They are also an excellent source of fiber. They're cheap and versatile, come in a variety of textures, and are packed with more nutrients per gram than any other food on Earth. Humans have eaten beans for at least 8,000 years; they're part of our culinary DNA. Even the Bible's book of Daniel (1:1-21) offers a two-week bean diet to make children healthier. The blue zones dietary average—at least a half cup per day—provides most of the vitamins and minerals you need. And because beans are so hearty and satisfying, they'll likely push less healthy foods out of your diet. Moreover, the high fiber content in beans helps healthy probiotics flourish in the gut.

Slash Sugar

Consume no more than seven added teaspoons a day. Centenarians typically eat sweets only during celebrations. Their foods have no added sugar, and they typically sweeten their tea with honey. This adds up to about seven teaspoons of sugar a day within the Blue Zones diets. The lesson to us: Enjoy cookies, candy, and bakery items only a few times a week and ideally as part of a meal. Avoid foods with added sugar. Skip any product where sugar is among the first five ingredients listed. Limit sugar added to coffee, tea, or other foods to no more than four teaspoons per day. Break the habit of snacking on sugar-heavy sweets. Let's face it: You can't avoid sugar. It occurs naturally in fruits, vegetables, and even milk. But that's not the problem. Between 1970 and 2000, the amount of added sugars in the food supply rose 25%. This adds up to about 22 teaspoons of added sugar that the average American consumes daily—insidious, hidden sugars mixed into sodas, yogurts, muffins, and sauces. Too much sugar in our diet has been shown to suppress the immune system, making it harder to fend off diseases. It also spikes insulin levels, which can lead to diabetes and lower fertility, make you fat, and even shorten your life. In the Blue Zones diet, people consume about the same amount of naturally occurring sugars as North Americans do, but only about a fifth as much added sugar. The key: People in the blue zones consume sugar intentionally, not by habit or accident.

Snack on Nuts

Eat two handfuls of nuts per day. The average amount that blue zones centenarians are eating equals about two ounces which is a handful. Here's how nuts are consumed in the various Blue Zones diets: Almonds in Ikaria and Sardinia, pistachios in Nicoya, and all nuts with the Adventists—all nuts are good. Nut-eaters on average outlive non-nut-eaters by two to three years. None of the blue zones centenarians have ever tried to live to 100. They don't count calories, take vitamins, weigh protein grams, or even read labels. They don't restrict their food intake—in fact, they all celebrate with food. As we have applied the wisdom of the world's Blue Zones diet to transform cities in the United State. We can create the same sort of culture here. It starts with food choices. Most of the blue zones residents have easy access to locally sourced fruits and vegetables—largely pesticide-free and organically raised. If not growing these food items in their own gardens, they have found places where they can purchase them, and more affordably than processed alternatives. They have incorporated certain nutritious foods into their daily or weekly meals—foods that often are not even found on the shelves of convenience stores or on the menus of fast-food restaurants across the country. They have inherited time-honored recipes or developed recipes on their own to make healthful foods taste good—a hugely important part of the Blue Zones diet, because if you don't like what you're eating, you're not going to eat it for very long. The particular foods important to blue zones centenarians vary from one culture to the next. What may be just as important, though, are the guidelines for food selection that we have developed after visiting numerous blue zones and finding the best ways to translate those values for North Americans. The findings here represent a long-term, statistical, and science-based study. We needed information that was not just anecdotal or based on interviews, visits in the kitchen, or shared meals with individual centenarians. We analyzed more than 150 dietary studies conducted in blue zones over the past century, and then we distilled those studies to arrive at a global average of what centenarians really ate. Here we provide some guidelines you can follow to eat a Blue Zones diet like they do and live to 100.

Sour on Bread

Replace common bread with sourdough or 100% whole wheat bread. Bread has been a staple in the human diet for at least 10,000 years. In three of the five blue zones diets, it is still a staple. While not typically used for sandwiches, it does make an appearance at most meals. But what people in blue zones are eating is a different food altogether from the bread that most North Americans buy. Most commercially available breads start with bleached white flour, which metabolizes quickly into sugar. White bread delivers relatively empty calories and spikes insulin levels. In fact, white bread (together with glucose) represents the standard glycemic index score of 100, against which all other foods are measured. Refined flour is not the only problem inherent to our customary white or wheat breads. Gluten, a protein, gives bread its loft and texture, but it also creates digestive problems for some people. Bread in the Blue Zones diet is different: either whole grain or sourdough, each with its own healthful characteristics. Breads in Ikaria and Sardinia, for example, are made from a variety of 100% whole grains, including wheat, rye, and barley—each of which offer a wide spectrum of nutrients, such as tryptophan, an amino acid, and the minerals selenium and magnesium. Whole grains all have higher levels of fiber than most commonly used wheat flours. Interestingly, too, barley was the food most highly correlated with longevity in Sardinia. Other traditional blue zones breads are made with naturally occurring bacteria called lactobacilli, which "digest" the starches and glutens while making the bread rise. The process also creates an acid—the "sour" in sourdough. The result is bread with less gluten than breads labeled "gluten-free" (and about one-thousandth the amount of gluten in normal breads), with a longer shelf life and a pleasantly sour taste that most people like. Most important, traditional sourdough breads consumed in Blue Zones diets lower the glycemic load of meals. That means they make your entire meal healthier, slower burning, easier on your pancreas, and more likely to make calories available as energy than stored as fat. Be aware that commercial sourdough bread found in the grocery store can be very different from traditional, real sourdough, and thus may not have the same nutritional characteristics. If you want to buy true sourdough bread, shop from a reputable—probably local— bakery and ask them about their starter. A bakery that cannot answer that question is probably not making true sourdough bread, and this should not be part of your Blue Zones diet.

whole food can say to be food made of a single ingredient, raw, cooked, ground, or fermented, and not highly processed. (Tofu is minimally processed, for example, while cheese doodles and frozen sausage dogs are highly processed.) Throughout the world's blue zones and their diets, people traditionally eat the whole food. They don't throw the yolk away to make an egg-white omelet, or spin the fat out of their yogurt, or juice the fiber-rich pulp out of their fruits. They also don't enrich or add extra ingredients to change the nutritional profile of their foods. Instead of vitamins or other supplements, they get everything they need from nutrient-dense, fiber-rich whole foods. And when they prepare dishes, those dishes typically contain a half dozen or so ingredients, simply blended together. Almost all of the food consumed by centenarians in the Blue Zones diet—up to 90%—also grows within a ten-mile radius of their home. Food preparation is simple. They eat raw fruits and vegetables; they grind whole grains themselves and then cook them slowly. They use fermentation—an ancient way to make nutrients bio-available—in the tofu, sourdough bread, wine, and pickled vegetables they eat. Eating only whole foods, people living in the blue zones rarely ingest any artificial preservatives. The foods they eat, especially the grains, are digested slowly, so blood sugar doesn't spike. Nutritional scientists are only just beginning to understand how all the elements from the entire plant (rather than isolated nutrients) work together synergistically to bring forth ultimate health. There are likely many thousands of phytonutrients—naturally occurring nutritional components of plants—yet to be discovered.

Blue Zone Diet and Workout

There is yet to be a practical evidence in the scientific literature to support the use of the Zone as an optimal muscle-building diet. In every case, the Zone may be one of the worst, for these reasons:

- The Zone supports a high protein to carbohydrate ratio. However, there is a negative correlation between the protein-carbohydrate ratio and serum testosterone levels (1). A diet of 10% protein has been associated with higher testosterone levels than a diet of 44% protein. The Zone recommends a diet of around 30% protein. Therefore, the Zone may result in lower serum T levels than other types of diets.

- If I remember correctly, Sears recommends about 1.0-1.6 g of carbohydrates for every gram of protein ingested, and about .4 g of fat for every gram of protein ingested. Sears also recommends ingesting about a gram of protein per lb. of bodyweight. Now, let's say I'm a 160 lb. person. This means I would have to ingest 160 g of protein a day, 256 g carbs, and 64 g of fat. This is a total 2240 kcal per day. This is not even close to enough calories to support building muscle while on a weight training program. Elite athletes need anywhere from 47 to 60 kcal/kg of bodyweight each day. For a 160 lb. person, this is 3418 to 4364 kcal per day. To increase muscle mass by 1 lb. a week, as much as 30 calories per lb. of bodyweight is needed. This is up to 4800 kcal per day. Sears's caloric recommendations don't even get much higher than the estimated REE for a 18-30-year-old male, which is 15.3 x wt.(kg) + 679. For our 160 lb. athlete, this is 1792 kcal per day.
- The protein recommendations of the Zone are too high. 1.5-2 g per kg of bodyweight is optimal for strength athletes if caloric intake matches energy expenditure.
- Sears's carbohydrate recommendations may be too low. A 65% carbohydrate diet has been found to result in better muscle gains than a 40% carbohydrate diet.
- There is no evidence in the scientific literature to support Sears's claim that the ratios he recommends will result in an optimal hormonal environment for muscle growth. The hormonal responses to food depend upon many factors, and not just the ratio of protein to carbohydrates to fats. The glycemic index of the foods ingested, the insulin sensitivity of the person eating the food, the amount of food ingested, etc., all are factors involved in the hormonal response to food.

When trying to build muscle, total caloric intake is always the most important factor. The ratio of nutrients ingested is secondary. The Zone diet does not allow for enough calories.

Does the Blue Zone Diet Work?

A collective document of the claimed centenarians found there may be some "fraud and error" in the statistics used to designate Blue Zones, DeRobertis says. "However, there is enough other substantiation for the health benefits of the diet and lifestyle modifications, even if the actual number of centenarians was not entirely accurate. These are still healthy lifestyle choices to aim to adapt that have been well documented," she says. "I think that people should review the findings of the Blue Zones and see what makes sense to incorporate into their lifestyle. People who make these changes usually lose weight, feel more connected to their community and feel less stress. There is no harm in adapting any of these principles. So yes, overall this is a lifestyle that I would recommend."

As with all eating plans, it's best to consult with a dietitian or nutritionist before making any changes to your diet. A specialist can help you pick the plan that will work best for your health history, lifestyle and, most importantly, what you like – and don't like – to eat. After all, no eating plan works if you don't enjoy it and stick with it. Not everyone agrees, of course. "I recommend some, but not all of the recommendations," says Aileen Birkitt, a registered dietitian and owner of Nutrition 4 You in North Kingstown, Rhode Island. She agrees with getting proper sleep and exercise, a greater focus on whole grain and plant-based foods and stopping eating when you are "almost full."

However, Birkitt disagrees with "the highly restrictive focus. It is very hard to avoid all sugar and processed foods in our society. Many times, the restriction and avoidance can lead to bingeing in those who are prone," she says. Birkitt also disagrees with avoiding dairy. "Dairy products are important as they provide calcium and protein to the diet. Someone who is not having these products needs to be sure to get enough calcium from other sources."

Birkitt also warns against the Blue Zone diet for anyone who has an eating disorder or a history of an eating disorder. "The avoidance of so many foods may cause someone to restrict foods that they might be able to eat in moderation, which might cause them to overeat from all the restricting and then feel guilt afterwards," she says.

Ultimately, as with all eating plans, it's best to consult with a dietitian or nutritionist before making any changes to your diet. A specialist can help you pick the plan that will work best for your health history, lifestyle and, most importantly, what you like – and don't like – to eat. After all, no eating plan works if you don't enjoy it and stick with it.

Sexual performance

sexual dysfunction is defined as a physical or psychological condition preventing a man from achieving sexual satisfaction and encompasses erectile dysfunction (ED), premature ejaculation, loss of libido, and hypogonadism. With increasing evidence about the impact of various diets on chronic diseases, there is a growing interest in establishing an association between various diets and men's health and sexual dysfunction. Erectile dysfunction appears to lessen in men adhering to the Mediterranean diet. Obese and overweight men who lose weight through low-fat, low-calorie diets seem to have improvements in their erectile function and testosterone levels.

The typical Mediterranean diet consists of fish, monounsaturated fats from olive oil, fruits, vegetables, nuts, legumes, and whole grains. The Mediterranean diet has been gaining increasing popularity during the past few decades given increasing health benefits demonstrated in randomized.

What does the Mediterranean diet do for sex?

For men with metabolic syndrome, Mediterranean diet helps to overcome erectile dysfunction (ED), or impotence. In fact, studies show that one-third of these men with ED cure their problem after following a Mediterranean-style diet, combined with exercise, for two years. Over 100 million men have ED worldwide.

No one knows with certainty how the Mediterranean Diet works, says Dr. La Puma, but because it reduces whole body inflammation and CRP (C-reactive protein) measurements, and improves endothelial (arterial lining) function, researchers think the Diet improves blood flow.

Belly fat, a big part of the metabolic syndrome, lowers testosterone levels. Losing that fat might improve androgen levels and improve the elasticity of blood vessels. By choosing foods on the Mediterranean Diet, it's possible to have better erections. "Less inflammation, better flow, better hormone levels, better erections," says Dr. La Puma.

Mediterranean Diet improves sexual desire

By consideration the specific dietary interventions in relation to erectile dysfunction, multiple Studies have looked specifically at the Mediterranean diet, which involves eating a diet high in Fruits and vegetables; limiting intake of refined sugars and processed foods; consuming more wholegrains, legumes, nuts, and seeds; replacing butter with healthful fats such as olive oil; and decreasing sodium intake by using more herbs and spices; limiting red meat consumption and increasing fish and poultry intake; and drinking red wine in moderation(optional).12 One study was conducted to determine whether the Mediterranean diet had any effects on Erectile dysfunction in men with the metabolic syndrome. 13 This group has multiple risk factors for erectile dysfunction, usually including diabetes, heart disease, and obesity. One-half of the Men participating in this study formed the control group, while the other half were placed on a two-year dietary intervention calling for participants to follow a Mediterranean diet. The intervention group received education on how to cut calories, set goals, and keep a food diary; participated in monthly small-group sessions; and received personalized diet advice based on three-day food records, which encouraged the consumption of fruits, vegetables, nuts, whole grains, and olive oil and discouraged the consumption of red or processed meat. 13 The intervention group took part in monthly sessions with a nutritionist during the first year and Then by monthly sessions during the second year. The men in the control group were given General diet education without an individualized program or regular meetings with a nutritionist. 13 At the end of two years, the men in the intervention group were eating more olive oil, nuts, Whole grains, fruits, and vegetables. They saw improvements in erectile dysfunction scores, but only one-third regained normal sexual function. The authors concluded, based on the Reduced levels of C-reactive protein, that the Mediterranean diet could be used to improve Vascular function, which can include erectile function. C-reactive protein is a marker of inflammation, which can negatively affect erectile function. 13 Since then, other studies have looked at the connection between the

Mediterranean diet and the incidence of erectile dysfunction. One study assessed the diets of men with type 2 diabetes and found that the greater their adherence to the Mediterranean diet, the lower the prevalence of erectile dysfunction. It's important to note, however, that the men who closely followed the Mediterranean diet also were more physically active and had lower BMIs, which could have Affected the prevalence of erectile dysfunction. 16 Esposito and colleagues reviewed similar studies and reached the same conclusion. They Determined that men who followed a dietary pattern high in fruits, vegetables, nuts, whole grains, and fish, and low in red and processed meat, and refined grains were less likely to experience erectile dysfunction. The Diet has been touted for its ability to reduce CVD, and improved vascular function leads to an improvement in blood flow to the penis. Another study concluded that patients with erectile dysfunction have high markers of oxidative Stress compared with those without dysfunction. 18 Oxidative stress causes inflammation, which Can lead to endothelial dysfunction. The Mediterranean diet naturally is high in antioxidants, which can reduce inflammation. Research indicates that men consuming the Mediterranean Diets have improvements in inflammatory markers and endothelial function.

Adherence to healthy diet promote healthy sex life

While nurturing relationships it is important to have a for a healthy sex life, what you eat plays an important role in your overall sexual health as well. Blue zones centenarians ate a predominantly plant-based diet for most of their lives. This is probably one of the reasons blue zones centenarians were able to enjoy good sex lives, even in their later years. Erectile dysfunction is an early indicator of poor vascular function, blood flow, and heart disease. The same clogged arteries that cause ED eventually also slow blood flow to the heart and the brain. The Massachusetts Male Aging Study found a direct connection between diet and ED. Men who ate plenty of fruits, vegetables, and whole grains, and who avoided red meat and highly processed foods were less likely to experience erectile dysfunction.

Effect of Mediterranean Diet on Hormonal imbalance

The Mediterranean Diet focuses on whole, real food with a balance of lean protein, complex carbohydrates and healthy fats. This makes it a great place to start when meal planning.

"Protein is necessary for muscle support and appetite control, and it is a healthy source of calories," shares Dr. Bitner. "Complex carbohydrates are necessary for energy as healthy calories and for replenishing liver glycogen as longer term energy stores for a work-out lasting more than 40 minutes."

So how does this relate to your hormones? Dr. Bitner adds that if a diet is high in simple sugar, calories not used immediately will be pushed into fat. This increases the risk of belly fat and pre-diabetes, which can leave even an athlete with low energy and poor ovarian function.

Effect of Diet on Estrogen Level

Estrogen dominance is a condition in which people have high levels of the sex hormone estrogen.   This condition has been linked to a variety of health issues, including certain types of breast cancer, ovarian cancer, and polycystic ovary syndrome (PCOS). Research shows that some dietary patterns are associated with higher levels of estrogen in the body, while other dietary patterns and specific foods may help decrease estrogen levels.

Estrogen is a hormone that plays critical roles in both female and male sexual function. In addition to being essential to reproductive health, estrogen is involved in many other systems in the body, including the immune, vascular, neuroendocrine, and skeletal systems.

The three main types of estrogen are estrone (E1), estradiol (E2), and estriol (E3). Estradiol is the most abundant and biologically active type of estrogen in women of reproductive age. The ovaries are the main producer of estradiol in the body.

Estradiol is found in both women and men, although women usually have much higher levels.   Although estrogen is an essential hormone, having too much estrogen can increase the risk of certain chronic diseases, including breast and ovarian cancer. This condition is formally known as estrogen dominance. Low estrogen can negatively affect health as well, but this article will mainly focus on estrogen dominance. Interestingly, research has shown that your diet and lifestyle can influence your estrogen levels. Some diets have been linked to healthy estrogen levels and a decreased risk of diseases associated with estrogen dominance. Meanwhile, others may increase estrogen levels.

Dietary choices can affect hormonal health and influence estrogen metabolism and excretion. Certain dietary patterns may lead to overweight and obesity, which may increase estrogen in the body.

Studies have found the Mediterranean diet is associated with healthy estrogen levels. It's rich in fish, vegetables, fruits, and legumes and restricts or limits foods associated with elevated estrogen, including processed and red meats and high fat processed foods.

An older study followed 115 women on a Mediterranean-style diet for 6 months. The diet was rich in plant protein and plant fats and low in animal proteins and animal fats. The women following the diet experienced a 40% decrease in total estrogen levels compared with women who made no dietary changes.

Fiber-rich diets like the Mediterranean diet tend to be high in phytoestrogens. These are molecules with estrogen-like activity found in certain foods like soy, legumes, nuts, grains, fruits, vegetables, and seeds. Phytoestrogens bind to estrogen receptors in cells and can have either antiestrogenic or estrogenic effects. For example, certain phytoestrogens compete with estrogen because they bind to estrogen receptors, blocking estrogen absorption.

For this reason, studies have shown that dietary patterns high in certain phytoestrogens may protect against hormone-sensitive cancers like certain breast cancers. High fiber, plant-based, and Mediterranean dietary patterns may help promote healthy estrogen regulation.

Tips for reducing estrogen levels

It's important to note that many factors beyond your diet, including your age and health status, can affect your body's hormone levels. This is why it's important to speak with your healthcare provider if you're concerned about estrogen dominance.

In general, the following tips may help promote healthy estrogen levels. Follow a fiber-rich diet. Studies have shown high fiber diets promote healthy estrogen levels. For example, increasing dietary fiber can help increase fecal excretion of estrogen, which may help control levels in the body. Limit certain animal products. Some studies have shown that red and processed meats may increase estrogen in the body, so limiting these foods may support estrogen regulation.

The Mediterranean diet, which is high in vegetables, whole grains, fruits, and legumes, has been associated with healthy estrogen levels and may help promote estrogen regulation Lose excess body fat. Losing excess body fat is an excellent way to reduce circulating estrogen. Plus, weight loss can help protect against many chronic diseases, including hormone-sensitive breast cancer.

Limit refined carbs and processed foods. Studies have associated Western dietary patterns rich in refined carbs and processed foods with elevated estrogen levels. Tip to considered in reducing estrogen level may include:

Exercise. In accordance with some research studies, exercise may help reduce circulating estrogen levels, promote healthy estrogen regulation, and protect against chronic diseases like breast cancer.

Limit alcohol intake. Some research shows that alcohol consumption can negatively affect hormones and may increase estrogen levels in some people.

Certain dietary patterns may help promote the healthy regulation of hormones, including estrogen. Some research has shown that diets rich in fiber and whole foods, such as the Mediterranean diet, are associated with optimal estrogen levels, while Western dietary patterns high in red and processed meats, sweets, and refined grains are associated with elevated estrogen levels.

Following a healthy diet and lifestyle is essential for hormonal health. However, many other factors can affect hormone levels, including age, medication use, and certain medical conditions.

Weight loss

The Mediterranean diet may also be helpful for people who are trying to lose weight. The authors of a 2016 review noted that people who were overweight or had obesity lost more weight on the Mediterranean diet than on a low-fat diet. The Mediterranean diet group achieved results that were similar to those of the participants on other standard weight loss diets.

Accountability

Losing weight can be challengingly frustrating, regardless if people want to lose a few pounds or 20. While weight loss usually requires dietary and lifestyle changes, as well as patience, some strategies may help people lose weight more quickly and safely.

A successfully weight lost requires a deliberate adherence to a healthy diet and regular exercise. Some popular diets are effective initially but may be challenging to maintain long-term. Individuals should personalize approaches to losing weight and consider their needs and lifestyle.

This book pictures a proper scientific study about how to lose weight successfully and safely. Using these tips may help someone lose 20 pounds or achieve their target weight, whatever that is. The Mediterranean diet encourages eating a variety of nutrient-rich foods and limits processed foods and added sugars, which are often high in calories. For this reason, pairing the Mediterranean diet with a healthy lifestyle could promote weight loss. One review of 5 studies found that the Mediterranean diet was as effective as other popular diets like the low carb diet for weight loss, resulting in up to 22 pounds (10 kg) of weight loss over 1 year. Likewise, a large study in over 32,000 people showed that long-term adherence to the Mediterranean diet was associated with a decreased risk of gaining weight and belly fat over 5 years

How to lose weight successfully and safely

More than 1 in 3 adults in the United States are overweight or have obesity. Experts agree that being overweight increases the risk of health conditions, including heart disease, diabetes, and high blood pressure.

To assess if they are overweight, a person can measure their waist circumference and calculate their body mass index (BMI). They can find out how much weight they need to lose to stay in healthy parameters.

According to the National Heart, Lung, and Blood Institute (NHLBI), people should initially aim to reduce their body weight by 10%. A sensible approach is to lose 1 to 2 pounds per week for 6 months. After that, someone can base their weight loss strategy on the results they have achieved. If someone has a lot of weight to lose, it may be wise to consult a doctor or registered dietitian to help them plan the best way to do this safely.

There are several diet and lifestyle approaches to losing weight. The following are tips that experts recognize as safe and effective ways to lose weight.

Reducing calories

The NHLBI suggest a person should reduce their daily calories by 500–1000 calories a day to lose weight. The National Institute of Diabetes and Digestive and Kidney Diseases (NIDDK) offer a Body Weight Planner to help someone make a personalized calorie and activity plan. Experts devised the planner according to how diet and exercise quantitatively influence someone's weight and help them maintain weight loss. Being mindful of portion size can help someone reduce their overall calorie intake. Eating mindfully and appreciating tastes and textures can help people reduce overeating. Avoiding eating meals in front of the TV or on the go can also help.

Avoiding refined carbohydrates and added sugars

Research suggests eating refined carbohydrates is associated with increased adiposity, insulin resistance, and obesity. Refined carbohydrates include foods made from white flour, such as white bread and pasta, pastries, and baked goods. To try and lose weight, people should consider choosing whole grain versions of carbohydrates and limiting their portion size. The Dietary Guidelines for Americans advise people to limit added sugars to less than 10% of their daily calories. Processed foods, sweetened drinks, and sauces often contain added sugars.

Eating more protein

A 2015 review indicates that higher-protein diets are beneficial for weight loss and satiety. The review suggests that the quantity of protein necessary to promote improved weight management is between 89–119 grams daily for women and 104–138 g daily for men.

Protein foods include:

- lean meat and poultry
- fish and seafood
- beans, lentils, and legumes
- tofu and plant-based proteins
- eggs and dairy products

Include healthy fats

A 2015 study indicates that reducing fats in the diet does not lead to more weight loss. The study also suggests that people eating a higher percentage of fats had slightly greater weight loss and better adherence compared to other diets. Another study indicates that people on weight loss diets that permit nuts, which contain healthy fats, lose more weight and comply better. Including smaller portions of healthful fats may help someone feel satisfied while they are losing weight. Doing this could help them avoid the temptation of sweet foods or refined carbohydrates.

Healthy fats include:

- extra virgin olive oil
- olives
- oily fish such as salmon, sardines, and mackerel

Exercising

A 2017 review concluded that consistently performing exercise for longer than the basic recommendations for health (150 min/week of moderate-intensity exercise) does appear to be more likely to contribute to weight loss and weight maintenance efforts over the long term. However, the same review recognized that variations in diet, BMI, and sex make conclusive recommendations more difficult. The study found that all types of exercise resulted in multiple health benefits for people with type 2 diabetes.

Another 2019 systematic review found strong evidence that people can maintain weight loss by increasing physical activity. People should do exercise that they enjoy and try different types to see what suits them. Types of activity could include walking or running, strength training, or yoga. Some people may prefer gym classes or team sports, and others may choose to follow instructions on a video class at home. unsalted and unflavored nuts such as almonds, walnuts, and Brazil nuts, seeds such as sunflower, hemp, pumpkin, and sesame seeds.

Increasing body mass

Athletes and fitness enthusiasts are constantly seeking new ways to boost their fitness performances and increase their muscle gains. They're trying to do this whilst remaining healthy and maintaining their general well-being. I believe that the best kind of diet is one rich in 'real,' whole foods. Nothing processed and very rarely packaged.

The only eating plan that supports this is the Mediterranean diet. There's close to 50 years of evidence backing its amazing benefits. Not only does the eating plan decrease your risk of diseases like heart disease, cancer,

Parkinson's, Alzheimer's and Type II Diabetes, but it even helps you live longer.

More importantly, the diet has a sustainable, flexible and enjoyable approach to food. Despite all else, switching from one fad diet to the next, can seriously mess with your hormones and stunt your fitness goals.

Mediterranean diet incorporates foods that provide you with the tools to boost your diet [longevity live] cardiovascular health, muscle growth and development. Not only does it promote nutrient-dense foods, but it even encourages physical exercise on a daily basis!

There are athletes who swear by it and have felt the physical advantages of following a Mediterranean meal plan. Even Cameron Van Der Burgh, a South African Olympic swimmer and champion, was recommended by experts to follow a Mediterranean diet after he had undergone a genetic testing.

In addition, oxidative stress and inflammation are both factors which will prevent you from reaching your true fitness potential. They can even prolong your recovery time. And since the Med-lifestyle reduces both inflammation and chronic disease... You are pretty much on your way to a life full of successful and rewarding gym experiences.

Body Transformation

You have the power to build a significant amount of muscle whilst on this diet. Not only this, but you can also boost diet [longevity live] your ability to endure high-intensity exercises. Mainly because you're consuming nutrient-dense food that has the ability to fuel your body for growth and recovery whilst maintaining heart health.

A very misleading notion has spread amongst the industry that protein is the only way to build muscle. Popular marketing tactics might have you believe this, but too much of anything is never a good thing. Overloading on one macronutrient is definitely not going to make the changes you want, happen.

The trick lies in this diet's limitless supply of vitamins, minerals and antioxidants. You can consume all the protein you want. But, without these crucial ingredients, you will never be able to achieve your best self.

If you are a strength athlete and wish to gain lean body mass or lose, do not doubt this diet, because you can do both with it. ManageYourMacros.Com explains that eating between 1.5-2.5g/kg of protein is more than enough for strength training athletes. And even though you might be skeptical because the Med-diet limits red meats, you can still get your iron and protein from other sources. So don't just introduce a ton of red meat when tweaking your meal plan.

These sources can include the following:

- fish and seafood
- beans
- poultry
- dairy
- eggs
- other plant-based sources.

In this way, you will fuel your body with plenty of necessary amino acids, vitamins and minerals. These are the ingredients that guarantee you a fully-functional, energetic and healthy body to reach optimal performance.

Moreover, many of the diets that are currently trending cut out major food groups, which can lead to a bunch of health problems because you're lacking in a specific nutrient. No matter how many crunches you do, you'll never get those washboard abs without these!

Adoption of plant-based diet

Research suggests that people can maintain their weight loss by increasing fruit and vegetable consumption. Data from three ongoing prospective cohort studies in the United States suggests that plant-based diets are associated with less weight gain over 4 years.

However, according to the study, an unhealthy plant-based diet does not have the same effect. The emphasis should be on whole foods that contain fiber. Fiber can positively affect satiety and the gut microbiome, leading to less adiposity, according to the study. Including more plant-based foods such as vegetables, fruits, and whole grains may help someone achieve their weight loss goals. People should try to avoid processed plant-based foods, as these can contain added sugars and unhealthy fats.

Getting adequate sleep

Research suggests that reduced sleep may lead to overeating and increased abdominal fat. Scientists believe short sleep duration over-activates the body's stress responses, which may lead to weight gain. People can try having a regular bedtime routine to promote sleep in the evening. Strategies such as avoiding screens, sleeping in a dark and quiet room, or exercising during the day may work for some people.

Increases sport activities

The Mediterranean diet (MD) is rich in vegetables, fruit, legumes, nuts, and cereals, with olive oil as the staple dietary fat. The typical MD includes moderate to high intake of fish, moderate intake of dairy products, and low consumption of meat products [1]. Adherence to the MD has been proven to have health benefits for adults, such as protection against cardiovascular disease [2], type 2 diabetes [3], and metabolic syndrome, and improving blood pressure, waist circumference, high-density lipoprotein cholesterol, triacylglycerol, and glucose concentration [4]. Despite these health benefits, adherence to the MD has been rapidly declining in Mediterranean countries [5] including Spain [6]. These countries are replacing the MD with a Western diet, which is rich in animal products, refined carbohydrates, and fat and lacking in consumption of fruit and vegetables. The benefits of physical exercise for health are well recognized [7]. An increase in physical activity has a significant role in the prevention of diseases such as cardiovascular disease, obesity, diabetes mellitus, cancer, depression, Alzheimer disease, arthritis, and osteoporosis [8]. Studies have shown an association between high levels of physical activity and Mediterranean diet adherence. Trends since the late 1990s also show adherence to be consistently higher in southern regions.

Effect of Mediterranean Diet on Disease prevention

Researchers have shown that adherence to this diet is associated with reduced risk of heart disease, certain cancers, diabetes, Parkinson's and Alzheimer's disease. In fact, evidence suggests that this diet is associated with a 20 percent reduced risk of death at any age.

The diet emphasizes whole grains, fruits, vegetables, beans, seeds, nuts, olive oil and fish. Herbs and spices are used instead of salt, and wine is consumed in moderation with meals. Red meats, processed foods, refined breads and food products high in saturated fats are visibly not part of this diet. A five year, rigorous 2013 study published in the New England Journal of Medicine was ended early because the benefits of the Mediterranean diet were so clear, that it became unethical to continue the study any longer, (since those in the control group were suffering). The magnitude of the diet's benefits surprised experts. Researchers found that switching to the Mediterranean diet could prevent about 30 percent of heart attacks, strokes and deaths from heart disease in people at high risk.

Now two independently published studies (May: JAMA Internal Medicine, and June: Bone and Mineral Research) lend even more support for this diet. The studies concluded that higher adherence to a Mediterranean diet is associated with a lower risk for fractures. In fact, the decrease in hip fracture incidence correlated closely with the degree of adherence to the Mediterranean diet. These results support that a healthy dietary pattern may play a key role in maintaining bone health. Since osteoporosis is the most common bone disease in the United States, tens of millions of people could be impacted by these findings. By 2020, it is estimated that one out of every two Americans over 50 will be at risk of developing osteoporosis of the hip. A Mediterranean diet can impact millions of lives by not only reducing fractures every year, but also by decreasing the incidence of prolonged pain, disability or even death.

Finally, other research has demonstrated that the Mediterranean diet might even reduce a senior's risk of developing muscle weakness and other signs of frailty by up to 70 percent. As we age, it is prudent to incorporate more vegetables, fruits, beans, nuts, fish, olive oil and whole grains into daily meals. The Blue Zones Project supports the

Mediterranean diet and lifestyle. There is already an abundance of proof supporting the Blue Zones way of life, and it appears that new evidence surfaces almost daily. Adopting the Mediterranean diet is a great way to start living healthier while eating fresh food in greater variety. The nutritional approach is very compatible with those who require low sodium, low fat or gluten-free diets. Given the flexibility and overwhelming positive evidence, the Mediterranean diet is a great option for anyone seeking health benefits for cardiovascular disease, bone health and longevity as a whole. So make it a priority to eat healthier and live longer.

Can adherence to Mediterranean Diet leads to Weight gain?

 when individuals take in more calories than they expend, the result will be weight gain. Given the growing incidence of obesity worldwide, however, it has become clear that this represents an over-simplification of a complex disease whose cure is more complicated than simply creating a caloric deficit. Physiologically, carbohydrate restriction, as opposed to a negative energy balance, is responsible for initiating the metabolic response to fasting.[2] The Atkins hypothesis is that dietary carbohydrate, particularly from simple sugars, causes hyperinsulinemia, leading to insulin resistance, obesity, and the metabolic syndrome. Excess carbohydrate prevents effective lipolysis with resulting lipo-genesis. Low carbohydrate diets reduce the dietary contribution to serum glucose thereby lowering insulin levels. Insulin is a potent stimulator of lipogenesis and inhibitor of lipolysis. Lowering insulin levels allows the utilization of stored body fat for energy. Severe carbohydrate restriction leads to a progressive depletion of glycogen stores eventually switching metabolism to lipolysis. With a reduction in dietary carbohydrate, there is a corresponding increase in dietary protein and fat. This leads to the production of ketones which act as an appetite suppressant and contribute to an overall voluntary caloric reduction.[3,4] It has been proposed that inefficient protein and fat oxidation leads to additional energy loss since more adenosine triphosphate (ATP) is required to oxidize these macronutrients.[5] Lipolysis is maintained despite excess calories because glycerol from fat is needed as a gluconeogenic precursor.[2] The carbohydrate level required to produce the metabolic shift from lipogenesis to lipolysis has been debated, but it is thought to be between 20 and 50 g of carbohydrate per day in the initial phases of the diet. This contrasts sharply with the typical carbohydrate content of the Western diet which often exceeds 300 g per day comprising large quantities of simple, rapidly hydrolyzed carbohydrates.(Clinical guide to popular diets)

Effects of the Mediterranean diet on Brain Function

Neurodegenerative diseases such as the most common form of dementia, Alzheimer's disease (AD), is an expanding issue worldwide with almost 50 million people suffering the disease (WHO, 2017), estimated to double in the next 20 years (Cheignon et al., 2018). As of yet, no treatment to cure the disease is available, forcing the need to investigate preventative strategies. For this reason, the Mediterranean diet has been highlighted for the beneficial effects on cardiovascular diseases and also more recently, cognitive deficits. Studies investigating the neurocognitive effects of the Medi are somewhat contradictive; also whether it is the whole diet with interacting nutrients, or single core nutrients present in the diet that drive the main beneficial effects, is still up for debate. This thesis will provide a general up to date review of the and discuss some nutrient compositions in the foods making up the diet; polyunsaturated fatty acids (PUFAs), antioxidants, polyphenols, and dietary fibers, due to the widely studied effects of these nutrients linked to cognitive decline, mood, and brain structure and function. The field of nutritional neuroscience is relatively new in the scientific community. The Journal of nutritional neuroscience has been active in almost two decades and aims to provide both basic and clinical research about nutrition and how it relates to the central nervous system and peripheral nervous system. It is an interdisciplinary field which might include the investigation of how dietary components such as protein, fats, and carbohydrates, or food supplements such as minerals and vitamins, affect the neurochemistry, neurobiology, and behavioral biology in humans and animals. The field can contribute by developing and investigating potential preventative strategies for diseases and conditions affecting individuals in today's society, for example AD and depression (Nutritional Neuroscience, 2018). In comparison, cognitive neuroscience is a somewhat more mature field which emerged in the late 1970s. Cognitive neuroscience combines the two disciplines of cognition; the process of knowing, and neuroscience; the study of how the nervous system is organized and functions. Nutritional neuroscience then touches and combines several disciplines to investigate how what we ingest then affects cognitive functions as well as brain structures.

When speaking about brain food we must not forget about one specific dietary regime which shows immense potential in maintaining and boosting brain functioning. This is the Mediterranean diet. Despite several differences between Mediterranean regions, they specific combination of foods make it so simple and yet so complicated at the same time. Yet this is exactly the perfect combination of macro and micronutrients, making it a number one choice for health and longevity. Health benefits of the MD go well beyond preventing cardiovascular disease, lower mortality and morbidity.

Similar characteristics of Blue Zones & the Mediterranean lifestyles

Obviously, the Mediterranean diet and the blue Zone Diet has a lot in common and can be replace by one over another. Thus, common features have be outline below:

- Meats are eaten only a few times a month in 3-4 ounce portions. Instead, the main protein sources come from beans & legumes, nuts, seeds, and fish. In the Blue Zones, beans are the foundation of most centenarian diets.
- The majority of foods consumed is plant-based; herbs and spices are used generously to season foods instead of salt; teas made from local herbs and water are the common most beverages; and fruit is frequently the after meal sweet.
- Movement is part of daily living activities. Instead of hitting the gym or pumping iron, the world's longest living people live in environments that involve lots of natural daily movement.
- Stress exists everywhere and can lead to chronic inflammation—one of the major contributors of chronic diseases. Stress-management routines vary but are deeply entrenched in the lifestyles leading to longevity.

- Social activities are important. Community participation and family connectedness among the generations have been shown to reduce morbidity and mortality rates in both the old and young

Introduction to keto Diet and Vegan Diet

Ketogenic" is a term for a low-carb diet (like the Atkins diet). The idea is for you to get more calories from protein and fat and less from carbohydrates. You cut back most on the carbs that are easy to digest, like sugar, soda, pastries, and white bread. Ketogenic diets are not just for losing weight. Many endurance athletes also turn to these very low-carb, high-fat diets to boost their performance But athletes involved in high-intensity, short-duration sports might see drops in performance while on a ketogenic diet, suggests new research.

Researchers from Saint Louis University tested the anaerobic exercise performance of 16 men and women following either a low-carbohydrate ketogenic diet or a high-carbohydrate diet for four days.

Carbs or low carbs for energy

Endurance athletes such as marathon runners and long-distance cyclists might fare better on a ketogenic diet than players who use short bursts of energy. Dr. Clifton Page, an assistant professor of orthopedics and family medicine at the University of Miami Miller School of Medicine, said "ketogenic diets appear to be beneficial for endurance athletes after a period of adaptation. Page said it can take several months on a ketogenic diet for the body to switch from using carbohydrates as its main energy source to using fats — the "adaptation period. To support the body as it makes the switch, ketogenic diets are very high in fats.

Zach Bitter, an ultra-marathoner and holder of the 100-mile American record and 12-hour world record, said "fat is always the primary macronutrient in my diet. It can reach as high as 70 percent when I am recovering from a big race or workout." But this doesn't mean ketogenic diets are high-protein diets.

In fact, eating too much protein can interfere with the production of ketones. These ketones are byproducts from the breakdown of fats and can be used as an alternative fuel source for the body when there isn't much glucose. Also, continuing to carb-load — such as with energy drinks and gels — can inhibit the body's switch to using ketones for energy.

"Metabolically, a high-carbohydrate diet locks an athlete into a dependence on glucose as the dominant fuel for exercise," said Jeff Volek, PhD, professor of human sciences and a registered dietitian at The Ohio State University and a leading researcher of carb-restricted diets. The body stores some glucose for later as glycogen. But Volek said the body has only enough glycogen to last about one day, or for just a few hours of hard exercise. So athletes on a high-carb diet need a steady intake of carbohydrates "to prevent this small carb fuel tank from running dry," he said.

Bitter said that since he switched to a ketogenic diet, he has been able to cut his in-race fueling by over 50 percent. He is quick to point out, though, that he doesn't "demonize carbs." But he tends to favor "low-glycemic sources of carbs in my meals when I do have them during peak training. People on the ketogenic diet performed more poorly at anaerobic exercise tasks than those eating more carbs.

Depending on the task, their performance was 4 to 15 percent lower than the high-carbohydrate group. The study was published last month in the Journal of Sports Medicine and Physical Fitness.

Study author Edward Weiss, PhD, associate professor of nutrition and dietetics at Saint Louis University, said that the results could make a big difference to athletes involved in sports that depend on short-burst anaerobic activities. This includes sprint-type activities that occur in soccer and basketball and also short, intense activities like the 100-meter sprint and the triple jump.

Weiss added that the study "probably also applies to many aerobic activities, as other studies have demonstrated that high-intensity aerobic exercise performance may be compromised by low-carb diets — including keto." In light of these results, he advised athletes to avoid these diets unless they have "compelling reasons for following a low-carb diet." While this is a small study and people were on the two diets for only a few days, a 2017Trusted Source review of previous research found similar early onset fatigue during short-duration activities while on a ketogenic diet.

For endurance athletes, long-term use of ketogenic diets may boost not only performance, but also overall health. "Keto-adaptation has enabled endurance athletes to set course and national records," said Volek. "And a growing number of military personnel are using ketosis to improve physical and cognitive performance and manage obesity, metabolic health, oxygen toxicity symptoms, and post-traumatic stress disorder."

Research — including a recent study by Volek — found that ketogenic diets may reduce body fat, type 2 diabetes, and metabolic syndrome. The last one is a group of conditions that includes high blood sugar and abnormal cholesterol levels. "More than half of adults have prediabetes or diabetes in the U.S., including athletes," said Volek. "A well-formulated ketogenic diet reverses the insulin-resistance phenotype more potently than any drug or lifestyle therapy." Bitter said he was attracted to a ketogenic diet not for the performance boost, but because during his training he would "wake up multiple times a night, experience big energy shifts throughout the day, and would get noticeable swelling in my legs and ankles after big workouts and races." The ketogenic diet helped with these symptoms. Not everyone thinks ketogenic diets are for every athlete.

"In many cases, you can still perform well at your chosen sport on very few carbs. But you are unlikely to perform at as high a level as you're accustomed to, and you're certainly not likely to perform your best," said Mike Israetel, PhD, head science consultant at Renaissance Periodization.

He added that your recovery after exercise will also be "significantly hampered, which will of course interfere with both performance and rates of improvement from training."

Page warned that research shows that "without long-term adaption to the ketogenic diet, an athlete could experience adverse effects including reduced muscle glycogen, hypoglycemia, and impaired athletic performance." If you do opt for a ketogenic diet, it's important to follow a plan designed by a nutritionist — or even work directly with someone experienced with these diets. While a lot of research focuses on the benefits of ketogenic diets for competitive athletes, weekend warriors and others may also benefit. "Recreational athletes tend to see more consistent benefits from adopting a ketogenic diet," said Volek. "In part because, on average, they have a greater emphasis on weight loss, metabolic and health benefits.   (Healthline.com)

How to Train Hard Enough on The Ketogenic Diet

With every workout, you are telling your cells what they need to adapt to. This is why it is always important to make your workouts more challenging little by little. If you don't, your muscles won't grow.

However, when you are first adapting to the ketogenic diet, you probably will not be able to work out with the same intensity as you did before. This happens because your body's ability to tap into glycolysis is severely impaired when it is first adapting to carbohydrate restriction. To understand what this means, we must dive deep into the cell where energy is formed.

There are three primary energy systems that your cells use to fuel themselves during exercise: the phosphagen system, the glycolytic pathway, and the aerobic system.

How to Build Muscle on the Keto Diet

Believe it or not, it's definitely possible to gain lean body mass while on the super-low-carb ketogenic diet. But it won't happen by accident! Here's what you need to do;

Keto and protein relationship

We know that getting adequate protein is crucial when it comes to building and maintain muscle mass. But as many lifters have discovered the hard way, that doesn't mean that eating more protein will automatically lead to more muscle growth. If only!

Still, someone who isn't following the ketogenic diet can keep piling on the protein without seeing much of a downside—except to their wallet and their digestion, perhaps. In the ketogenic diet, however, eating wildly excessive amounts of protein can actually kick you out of ketosis. This is why the ketogenic diet is usually considered to be a "moderate" protein diet, not a high-protein diet.

So, what's "moderate?" As explained in the article "Ketogenic Diet: Your Complete Meal Plan and Supplement Guide," an effective ketogenic diet should include 15-20 percent of total calories from protein. This is quite low compared to the 30-40 percent of calories from protein touted by most online nutrition calculators in the bodybuilding community when you set your goal as "muscle growth."

But get this: A study published in the Journal of Sports Sciences found that consuming 0.6-0.8 grams of protein (evenly distributed between 3-4 meals while also in a calorie surplus) was adequate to optimize levels of muscle protein synthesis. Devoting 15-20 percent of your calories to protein is enough to get you to that threshold.

Tempted to go higher, like the classic 1 gram per pound of body weight or higher? That's a classic mistake for aspiring ketogenic dieters, and here's why: When your body is deprived of carbs, eating too much protein can lead to some of the protein being converted into glucose, which knocks you out of ketosis. The result is you end up feeling like crap and dragging through your workouts because your body gets just enough carbs to stay carb-adapted, but without converting fully to the fat-burning benefits true ketosis has to offer!

Afraid of your gains melting away? Don't be. When you follow a ketogenic diet, the prolonged absence of carbohydrates leads to an increased production in ketones, which are a byproduct of fat breakdown. One unique benefit of having elevated levels of ketones in your blood is that they're muscle-sparing.

One ketone, called beta-hydroxybutyrate (BHB), has even been shown in a small, human study to have a positive impact on muscle growth, specifically leading to a decrease in leucine oxidation while also promoting protein synthesis. And when it comes to muscle growth, every little bit helps!

Still, it's understandable to be hesitant about potentially cutting back on protein. Here are three ways to make sure that you're getting the most out of every gram in your diet while following the ketogenic diet

High quality protein: A high-quality protein source is one that contains all nine essential amino acids and is specifically rich in the key muscle-building amino acid leucine. Lower-quality proteins, like grains and legumes, aren't usually on the menu for the ketogenic diet anyway. And the animal-based protein sources that are typical to keto are all fantastic sources of complete, high-quality protein.

Solid choices include eggs (both yolk and white), whole-fat milk, Greek yogurt, cheese, chicken, turkey, pork, beef, lamb, fish, and seafood. As much as possible, get your protein from these sources, and you'll give your body more of the amino acids it needs to preserve and add lean muscle mass.

Protein Timing: Research in recent years has reinforced the idea that it's not just how much protein you eat in a day that matters, but also when you eat it—or more specifically, how you space it out across the day. To receive maximal benefit from the protein you consume, you should eat a specific amount of high-quality protein—enough to reach what is known as the "leucine threshold"—every few hours. And doing so consistently throughout the day, day after day and week after week, will yield some fantastic muscle-growth results—assuming you're also in an overall calorie surplus and training hard consistently.

But once you've met this threshold at a meal—which is 25-35 grams of protein per meal for most individuals—there's no added muscle-building benefit. This is especially true if it will kick you out of ketosis. Keep it simple: Focus on eating 3-4 meals per day, each with a fairly consistent amount of protein, so that you can reach the leucine threshold at each meal.

Calorie Surplus: Most people embark on a ketogenic journey to lose body fat. But if your body composition goal is to build muscle, a calorie deficit will not help you accomplish it. No matter what type of diet you follow, one thing that is always true is that your muscles need calories to grow! Remember, the study mentioned earlier determined that consuming moderate protein was sufficient, provided the subjects spread out their meals and ate in a caloric surplus. That last part is key! While you're doing keto, do your best to at least eat a maintenance number of calories. But if you're looking to grow, definitely count calories to the best of your ability to make sure you're in a surplus.

Vegan diet

Vegan or plant-based diet excludes all animal products, including meat, dairy, and eggs. When people follow it correctly, a vegan diet can be highly nutritious, reduce the risk of chronic diseases, and aid weight loss. However, people eating only plant-based foods need to be more aware of how to obtain certain nutrients, including iron, calcium, and vitamin B-12, that usually come from an omnivorous diet.

Vegan diets tend to include plenty of fruits, vegetables, beans, nuts, and seeds. Eating a variety of these foods will provide a wide range of important vitamins, minerals, healthful fats, and protein. A healthy, plant-based diet aims to maximize consumption of nutrient-dense plant foods while minimizing processed foods, oils, and animal foods (including dairy products and eggs). It encourages lots of vegetables (cooked or raw), fruits, beans, peas, lentils, soybeans, seeds, and nuts (in smaller amounts) and is generally low fat. Leading advocate in the field have varying opinions as to what comprises the optimal plant-based diet .It was recommended that allowing animal products such as egg whites and skim milk in small amounts for reversal of disease. The director of the cardiovascular prevention and reversal program at the Cleveland Clinic Wellness Institute Esselstyn recommends completely avoiding all animal-based products as well as soybeans and nuts, particularly if severe coronary artery disease is present. Despite these smaller differences, there is evidence that a broadly defined plant-based diet has significant health benefits. It should be noted that the term plant-based is sometimes used interchangeably with vegetarian or vegan. Vegetarian or vegan diets adopted for ethical or religious reasons may or may not be healthy. It is thus important to know the specific definitions of related diets and to ascertain the details of a patient's diet rather than making assumptions about how healthy it is. The following is a brief summary of typical diets that restrict animal products. A key distinction is that although most of these diets are defined by what they exclude, the plant-based diet is defined by what it includes.

Vegan (or total vegetarian): Excludes all animal products, especially meat, seafood, poultry, eggs, and dairy products. Does not require consumption of whole foods or restrict fat or refined sugar. Raw food, vegan: Same exclusions as veganism as well as the exclusion of all foods cooked at temperatures greater than 118°F. The major types of vegan include:

Lacto-vegetarian: Excludes eggs, meat, seafood, and poultry and includes milk products.

Ovo-vegetarian: Excludes meat, seafood, poultry, and dairy products and includes eggs.

Lacto-ovo vegetarian: Excludes meat, seafood, and poultry and includes eggs and dairy products.

Vegan Diet is closely like Mediterranean Diet, thus Similar to whole-foods, plant-based diet but allows small amounts of chicken, dairy products, eggs, and red meat once or twice per month. Fish and olive oil are encouraged. Fat is not restricted. Whole-foods, plant-based, low-fat: Encourages plant foods in their whole form, especially vegetables, fruits, legumes, and seeds and nuts (in smaller amounts). For maximal health benefits this diet limits animal products. Total fat is generally restricted.

Health Benefits of Vegan Diet

Reduces risk of heart disease

In some previous Studies it has been proven that vegans have better heart health and lower odds of having certain diseases. Those who skip meat have less of a chance of becoming obese or getting heart disease, high cholesterol, and high blood pressure. Vegans are also less likely to get diabetes and some kinds of cancer, especially cancers of the GI tract and the breast, ovaries, and uterus in women.

A large scale 2019 study has linked a higher intake of plant-based foods and lower intake of animal foods with a reduced risk of heart disease and death in adults. Animal products — including meat, cheese, and butter — are the main dietary sources of saturated fats. According to the

American Heart Association (AHA), eating foods that contain these fats raises cholesterol levels. High levels of cholesterol increase the risk of heart disease and stroke. Plant foods are also high in fiber, which the AHA link with better heart health. Animal products contain very little or no fiber, while plant-based vegetables and grains are the best sources.

In addition, people on a vegan diet often take in fewer calories than those on a standard Western diet. A moderate calorie intake can lead to a lower body mass index (BMI) and a reduced risk of obesity, a major risk factor for heart disease.

Lower cancer risk

According to a 2017 review, eating a vegan diet may reduce a person's risk of cancer by 15%. This health benefit may be due to the fact that plant foods are high in fiber, vitamins, and phytochemicals — biologically active compounds in plants — that protect against cancers.

Research into the effects of diet on the risk of specific cancers has produced mixed results. However, the International Agency for Research on Cancer report that red meat is "probably carcinogenic," noting that research has linked it primarily to colorectal cancer but also to prostate cancer and pancreatic cancer.

The agency also report that processed meat is carcinogenic and may cause colorectal cancer. Eliminating red and processed meats from the diet removes these possible risks.

Promote weight loss

People on a vegan diet tend to have a lower body mass index (BMI) than those following other diets. The researchers behind a 2015 study reported that vegan diets were more effective for weight loss than omnivorous, semi-vegetarian, and pesco-vegetarian diets, as well as being better for providing macronutrients. Many animal foods are high in fat and calories, so replacing these with low calorie plant-based foods can help people manage their weight. It is important to note, though, that eating lots of processed or high fat plant-based foods — which some people refer to as a junk food vegan diet — can lead to unhealthful weight gain.

Lower risk of type 2 diabetes

According to a large 2019 review, following a plant-based diet can reduce the risk of type 2 diabetes. The research linked this effect with eating healthful plant-based foods, including fruits, vegetables, whole grains, nuts, and legumes.

Nutrients to consider on a vegan diet

A vegan diet removes some sources of nutrients from the diet, so people need to plan their meals carefully to avoid nutritional deficiencies. People may wish to talk to a doctor or dietitian ahead of adopting a vegan diet, especially if they have existing health conditions.

Key nutrients low in a vegan diet

Vitamin B-12:

 Vitamin B-12 is mainly present in animal products. It protects the nerves and red blood cells. Plant-based sources of this vitamin include fortified cereals and plant milks, nutritional yeast, and yeast spreads. Read more about vegan sources of vitamin B-12.

Iron:

Iron is important for blood health. Beans and dark leafy greens are good sources. Find out more about iron-rich vegan foods.

Calcium:

Calcium is crucial for bone health. Eating tofu, tahini, and leafy greens will help keep calcium levels up. Learn about calcium-rich plant-based foods.

Vitamin D:

Vitamin D protects against cancer and some chronic health conditions, and it helps strengthen the bones and teeth. Regularly eating vitamin D-fortified foods and spending time in the sun can boost vitamin D levels.

Omega-3 fatty acids:

Important for heart, eye, and brain function, there are three types of omega-3 fatty acid: EPA, DHA, and ALA. Walnuts and flaxseeds are good sources of ALA, but seaweeds and algae are the only plant sources of EPA and DHA. Read about how to get omega-3 as a vegan.

Zinc:

Zinc is important for the immune system and the repair of DNA damage. Beans, nutritional yeast, nuts, and oats are high in zinc. Read about zinc-rich vegan foods.

Iodine:

Iodine is important for thyroid function. Plant-based sources include seaweeds and fortified foods.

Role of Vegan diet in present sport

Vegan diets are booming in the mainstream and in sport. From current sporting success all the way back to ancient times, it is evident that vegans can win races up to professional levels and even break records. However, despite the sound health benefits of vegan diets, vegan athletes are frequently faced with prejudice on unsubstantiated grounds. Therefore, this review considers the various advantages of the vegan diet for young and competitive athletes. It encompasses early studies and compares the potential benefits and risks by looking at the quality of animal and plant protein. The knowledge that vegan diets are compatible with sports performance has the potential to encourage athletes and their families, coaches, and experts in health and sports to be more open-minded when an athlete expresses his/her desire to adopt a vegan diet.

A short outline of the future perspectives of research needed is given below:

Nutrient considerations and recommendations

Energy and macronutrients

Energy:

Meeting energy needs is a nutrition priority for all athletes (Thomas et al., 2016). Inadequate energy intake negates the benefits of training, compromises performance and may result in health complications that include a loss of muscle mass and/or bone density, and an increased risk of fatigue, injury and illness. Energy requirements vary among individual athletes according to the specific sport, intensity and periodized training activities at which athletes participate (which are likely to vary from day to day and across the season). Other influencing factors include sex, age and body composition. Some vegetarian and vegan athletes may not meet their energy needs due to the high-fiber and low-energy density of plant-based diets combined with elevated energy needs and/or hectic schedules that prohibit adequate time to eat. Athletes with high-energy needs should be encouraged to eat frequent meals and snacks (i.e., ~5-8 meals/snacks/day) and adequately plan so food and snacks are readily available. For example, snacks or mini-meals packed in a gym bag, back pack or kept in a locker or desk drawer provide readily available food energy. Selection of energy-dense foods and limiting of fiber-rich foods may also help meet energy needs. For example, replacing some whole fruit servings with fruit juice and consuming one-third to one-half of grains, cereals and breads as less processed sources, such as white rice or sourdough bread rather than brown rice or whole wheat bread will reduce excessive fiber intake and the early onset of satiety (Grandjean, 1987; Larson-Meyer, 2007). In contrast, other vegetarian athletes may require lower energy intakes to promote a slow and sustained weight reduction for health and/or performance reasons. These athletes may benefit from an emphasis on the selection of whole, unprocessed foods to promote satiety and help in achievement of a healthy body weight.

Many publicly available food guidance systems geared at athletes, vegetarians or the general public may be useful for helping educate vegetarian and vegan athletes on healthy eating patterns that meet energy needs. These include USDA's MyPlate, which has adjustments for energy requirements and tips for vegetarian diets (United States Department of Agriculture), the United States Olympic Committee Sports Dietitians Athlete's Plates (which are based on training phase and easily adopted to vegetarian patterns) (The United States Olympic Committee Sports Dietitians; The University of Colorado Sports Nutrition Graduate Program, 2006), and the guidelines developed specifically for vegetarian athletes (Larson-Meyer, 2007). Vegetarian or vegan-specific eating plans, such as The Vegetarian Resource Groups "My Vegan Plate"(Vegetarian Resource Group, 2011), may also provide a useful framework if the number of servings is appropriately adjusted to meet the higher energy demands of many athletes.

Carbohydrate:

Carbohydrates are an important component of an athlete's diet and should make up the bulk of their energy intake. Carbohydrate ingestion is essential for optimal performance during prolonged moderate- to high-intensity exercise lasting longer than ~90 min and during intense intermittent activities, which are typical of many team sports (Burke et al., 2011, Thomas et al., 2016). Carbohydrates are also necessary for glycogen repletion following exercise and to ensure adequate adaptation to training. The amount of carbohydrates that active vegetarians need to ingest varies, depending on sport, intensity, and body mass (BM). The current carbohydrate recommendations are 5-10 g carbohydrate/kg BM/day for most athletes performing moderate- to high-intensity exercise of ~1-3 h/day (Thomas et al., 2016). Lower intakes of 3-5 g/kg BM are suggested for athletes performing low-intensity or skill-based training while higher requirements of 8-12 g/kg BM are recommended during extreme endurance training(Burke et al., 2011; Thomas et al., 2016). Although the typical vegetarian diet is packed with carbohydrate, the importance of achieving adequate carbohydrate is emphasized here in light of the recent popularity of lower carbohydrate diets that also may be "attractive" to certain vegetarian athletes. Vegetarian athletes, like all athletes, should be educated on the proper types of carbohydrates to eat surrounding an exercise session.

Protein:

Protein requirements vary according to training level and type of activity. An athlete undergoing intense training will need more protein than a person who is recreationally active and exercises moderately several days a week. The US Recommended Dietary Allowance (RDA) of 0.8 g protein/kg BM/day should meet the needs of most people who exercise at a light to moderate intensity most days of the week. Athletes who train at higher intensities generally need more protein. Emerging research on protein requirements of athletes suggests that dietary protein interacts with exercise providing not only a substrate for the synthesis of contractile, structural and metabolic proteins but also a trigger for muscle protein synthesis (Phillips & van Loon, 2011; Thomas et al., 2016). The current protein intake recommendations for athletes is 1.2-2.0 g protein/kg BM/day which is recommended to support metabolic adaptation, repair, remodeling, and protein turnover.

There is little evidence to suggest that the protein requirements for athletes following vegetarian diets are different from those following omnivorous diets, particularly given the large range suggested by the current protein requirements for athletes. To ensure adequate protein intake, vegetarian athletes should be encouraged to consume a variety of plant-based protein-rich foods and ensure adequate energy intake. Good sources of plant-based and vegetarian proteins (>7 g protein/serving), however, it is important to remember that all grains, cereals and starchy vegetables also contribute small amounts of protein (2-3 g/serving). Vegetarians do not need to consume specific combinations of plant-based protein at each meal but should consume a variety of protein sources spread throughout the day. One exception may be in the post-exercise period for athletes undergoing intense muscle-based training where a certain concentration of serum leucine and ~10 g of essential acids may be necessary to optimize muscle protein synthesis in the immediate post-exercise period. Many plant proteins including legumes are leucine-rich, albeit not as well absorbed as whey protein. Furthermore, usual culinary combinations of protein such as beans and rice, beans and nuts/seeds (e.g., in hummus) or a peanut butter sandwich tend to be complementary.

Fat:

Fat intake guidelines for athletes should be in accordance with public health guidelines, and be individualized based on training and body composition goals (Thomas et al., 2016). Dietary fat is necessary in order to provide energy, elements of cell membranes and essential fatty acids, and to aid in the absorption of fat-soluble vitamins. Fat stored within active muscle and adipocytes is used as a substrate during prolonged exercise of moderate-intensity and during low-level activity. Thus, dietary sources of essential fatty acids should be emphasized to meet intake recommendations and saturated fat be limited to less than 10% of total energy intake (U.S. Department of Health and Human Services and U.S. Department of Agriculture, 2011). Both chronic low-fat intake below 20% of energy and strategies which promote low-carbohydrate, high-fat diets for purported performance benefits are discouraged (Thomas et al., 2016). Although extremely low-fat vegan diets (< 10% energy from fat) are recommended for the prevention and treatment of cardiovascular disease and diabetes, such diets are too restrictive for athletes undergoing intense training regimens. The currently popular trend of fat adaptation to enhance fat oxidation via extremely high-fat, low-carbohydrate diets has been shown to down regulate carbohydrate metabolism and compromise performance during the high-intensity exercise bouts that are common in most sports.

Vegetarian and vegan athletes can ensure that fat intake is appropriate within the guidelines through judicious selection of plant-based sources and low- or full-fat dairy products, as desired. In general, however, the vegetarian diet is rich in omega-6 polyunsaturated fatty acids but limited in omega-3 fatty acids. Lacto-ovo diets can also provide excessive saturated fat if intake of animal-derived fats including cheese and other full-fat dairy products and eggs are consumed regularly. Because omega-3 fatty acids may be important for inflammatory modulation, vegetarian athletes may benefit from intentional selection of omega-3 rich foods in place of some or in addition to omega-6 rich oils (corn, cotton seed, sunflower and safflower). Even though endogenous elongation of alpha-linolenic acid (ALA) to eicosapentaenoic acid (EPA) is inefficient and influenced by health status, sex, age and diet composition (its conversion is increased when omega-6 concentrations are low), evidence suggests that omega-3 needs can be met with ALA alone. Endogenous synthesis of EPA and Docohexanoic acid (DHA) from ALA appears to be sufficient to maintain long-term stable concentrations in vegetarians. Vegetarian athletes may also consider DHA-rich microalgae supplements, which are well-absorbed and increase DHA and EPA concentrations in blood. Athletes habitually obtaining more than 10% of energy from saturated fat should replace some servings of full-fat dairy and/or eggs with plant-based sources.

Vitamins and Minerals:

Vitamins and minerals are an essential part of the diet of all athletes. Vegetarian athletes may need to pay particular attention to a handful of nutrients which are either found less abundantly in vegetarian foods or are less well absorbed from plant compared to animal sources. These nutrients include iron, zinc, calcium, vitamin D, iodine and some of the B-vitamins (B-12 and riboflavin). Other nutrients including potassium, magnesium, folate, vitamins A, C, E and K are typically provided abundantly by a well-balanced vegetarian diet.

Iron:

Iron intake can be a concern for vegetarian athletes, particularly female athletes. Non-heme iron (plant-based iron) is best absorbed with foods that contain ascorbic acid (i.e., citrus fruit or juice, tomatoes and melon) and other organic acids and is inhibited by plant phytates, polyphenolics, tannins in tea, cocoa and coffee, soy and dairy protein, and foods with high concentrations of calcium, zinc or other divalent minerals. Cooking with iron cookware also boosts iron content, particularly when the foods are slightly acidic (i.e., tomato sauce). If iron status is a concern, the sports dietitian or physician should assess whether iron supplementation is needed. High-dose iron supplements should not be taken unless iron deficiency is present, as it may interfere with absorption of other minerals and can lead to excess iron stores in individuals at risk for hemochromatosis.

Zinc:

Like iron, suboptimal zinc status may be somewhat prevalent in certain athletes, including female athletes and athletes following vegan and vegetarian diets. In vegetarians, lower zinc status may be attributed to the selection of zinc-poor foods or the reduced bioavailability of zinc from plant compared to animal foods. Vegetarians who eat a varied and well-balanced diet that contains many zinc-rich plant food including legumes and whole grains are likely to achieve adequate zinc status without dietary supplementation. Similar to iron, organic acids such as citric, malic and lactic acids can enhance zinc absorption to some extent, whereas food preparation techniques such as soaking, sprouting of beans, grains, nuts and seeds, and leavening akee is a concern for vegan athletes and vegetarians who consume minimal dairy products. Although it is possible for vegetarians, including vegans, to meet recommendations for calcium, judicious selection of well-absorbable sources of calcium along with possible use of calcium-fortified foo The calcium bioavailability of most of these plant foods is as good as or better than cow's milk, which has a fractional absorption of 32% . Exceptions include spinach, chard, beet greens and rhubarb, which have a low bioavailability (< 5-8%) due to the high oxalate content of these foods. Vitamin D, which aids in calcium absorption, may also be a concern for some athletes due to limited sun exposure and/or reduced intake of Vitamin D-containing foods. While vegetarians and vegans may be at additional risk due to lower dietary intake, factors such as skin pigmentation, sun exposure intensity and dietary supplementation are more important predictors of vitamin D status than is intake from food sources. Vitamin D requirements can be met by exposing arms, legs, and abdomen and back (i.e., in shorts and a sports bra) to noontime sunlight for ~10-30 min several times a week depending on skin pigmentation. Supplementation (1,000-2,000 IU/day) may be beneficial, especially for athletes living at extreme latitudes (> 35 degrees north or south latitude), who train primarily indoors, use excessive sunscreen or have excess body fat, dark pigmented or very fair skin or photosensitivity. Vegans can be directed to look for vitamin D-3 derived from lichen, rather than lanolin, and D-2 produced from irradiation of yeast ergosterol. Research has suggested, however, that vitamin D-2 may be less effective than vitamin D-3 when taken in higher doses (> 4,000 IU).

Iodine:

Poor iodine status is common in many vegans and vegetarians who do not consume table salt (typically fortified with iodine) or sea vegetables, or consume plant foods grown in iodine-poor soil. There is also some evidence that iodine is lost in sweat which may place athletes who sweat heavily at additional risk for suboptimal status. Adequate iodine status can be assured by encouraging athletes to use iodized salt in cooking and salting foods (1/2 teaspoon or 3 g provides close to the RDA and 1,180 mg sodium) along with appropriately reducing intake from processed foods. Sea salt, gourmet salts, most salty seasonings (tamari, soy sauce) and most sodium-containing processed foods are not iodized.

Vitamin B-12 and Riboflavin:

Athletes who follow vegan or near vegan diets are at risk for low vitamin B12 status (Pawlak et al., 2013), which is found exclusively in animal products (Melina et al., 2016). Vegan athletes should consume vitamin B-12 fortified foods daily or take a vitamin B-12 containing supplement or multivitamin. Vegetarian athletes should also consider taking a supplemental source if their intake of dairy products and/or eggs is limited. Riboflavin may also be a concern to vegan and vegetarians who limit intake of dairy (Herrmann & Geisel, 2002) and possibly also restrict energy intake.

Things to consider before going vegan or keto:

Before deciding to do any diet, ask yourself why you are going on the diet. Is it for nutritional, environmental or ethical reasons? Are you trying to lose weight or improve a health condition like diabetes or cholesterol? This can help guide you toward the diet best suited for you and your goals. Check with your doctor to see if it is healthy for you given your medical history and nutrient status to start eating vegan or keto.

If choosing a diet for weight loss, ask yourself, "What plans have I tried in the past, and why did they fail?" Were the food choices too restrictive? Did you lose motivation? Were you always hungry? Understanding what works and does not work for you and talking to your health care providers, including your physician and a dietitian, to determine which diet is best for you based on your goals, will be most successful.

Review your current lifestyle and how much time you have to devote to food preparation or calculating macronutrients like carbs in your diet. Do you eat outside the home a lot? Does your schedule allow for food preparation? It's not impossible to do vegan or keto while traveling or eating out, but (as with most diets) preparation and planning are key— as is working with a professional who can guide you.

Healthy diet

Consuming a healthy diet throughout the life-course helps to prevent malnutrition in all its forms as well as a range of noncommunicable diseases (NCDs) and conditions. However, increased production of processed foods, rapid urbanization and changing lifestyles have led to a shift in dietary patterns. People are now consuming more foods high in energy, fats, free sugars and salt/sodium, and many people do not eat enough fruit, vegetables, and other dietary fiber such as whole grains.

The exact make-up of a diversified, balanced and healthy diet will vary depending on individual characteristics (e.g. age, gender, lifestyle and degree of physical activity), cultural context, locally available foods and dietary customs. However, the basic principles of what constitutes a healthy diet remain the same.

A healthy diet helps to protect against malnutrition in all its forms, as well as noncommunicable diseases (NCDs), including such as diabetes, heart disease, stroke and cancer. Unhealthy diet and lack of physical activity are leading global risks to health. Healthy dietary practices start early in life – breastfeeding fosters healthy growth and improves cognitive development, and may have longer term health benefits such as reducing the risk of becoming overweight or obese and developing NCDs later in life. Energy intake (calories) should be in balance with energy expenditure. To avoid unhealthy weight gain, total fat should not exceed 30% of total energy intake. Intake of saturated fats should be less than 10% of total energy intake, and intake of trans-fats less than 1% of total energy intake, with a shift in fat consumption away from saturated fats and trans-fats to unsaturated fats , and towards the goal of eliminating industrially-produced trans-fats. Limiting intake of free sugars to less than 10% of total energy intake is part of a healthy diet. A further reduction to less than 5% of total energy intake is suggested for additional health benefits. Keeping salt intake to less than 5 g per day (equivalent to sodium intake of less than 2 g per day) helps to prevent hypertension and reduces the risk of heart disease and stroke in the adult population. WHO Member States have agreed to reduce the global population's intake of salt by 30% by 2025; they have also agreed to halt the rise in diabetes and obesity in adults and adolescents as well as in childhood overweight by 2025.

Maintaining a healthy diet

Fruit and vegetables

Eating at least 400 g, or five portions, of fruit and vegetables per day reduces the risk of NCDs (2) and helps to ensure an adequate daily intake of dietary fiber.

Fruit and vegetable intake can be improved by:

- always including vegetables in meals;
- eating fresh fruit and raw vegetables as snacks;
- eating fresh fruit and vegetables that are in season; and
- eating a variety of fruit and vegetables.

Fats

Reducing the amount of total fat intake to less than 30% of total energy intake helps to prevent unhealthy weight gain in the adult population. Also, the risk of developing NCDs is lowered by:

- reducing saturated fats to less than 10% of total energy intake;
- reducing trans-fats to less than 1% of total energy intake; and
- replacing both saturated fats and trans-fats with unsaturated fats (2, 3) – in particular, with polyunsaturated fats.

Fat intake, especially saturated fat and industrially-produced trans-fat intake, can be reduced by:

- steaming or boiling instead of frying when cooking;

- replacing butter, lard and ghee with oils rich in polyunsaturated fats, such as soybean, canola (rapeseed), corn, safflower and sunflower oils;
- eating reduced-fat dairy foods and lean meats, or trimming visible fat from meat; and
- limiting the consumption of baked and fried foods, and pre-packaged snacks and foods (e.g. doughnuts, cakes, pies, cookies, biscuits, and wafers) that contain industrially produced trans-fats.

Salt, sodium and potassium

Most people consume too much sodium through salt (corresponding to consuming an average of 9–12 g of salt per day) and not enough potassium (less than 3.5 g). High sodium intake and insufficient potassium intake contribute to high blood pressure, which in turn increases the risk of heart disease and stroke.

Reducing salt intake to the recommended level of less than 5 g per day could prevent 1.7 million deaths each year.

People are often unaware of the amount of salt they consume. In many countries, most salt comes from processed foods (e.g. ready meals; processed meats such as bacon, ham, and salami; cheese; and salty snacks) or from foods consumed frequently in large amounts (e.g. bread). Salt is also added to foods during cooking (e.g. bouillon, stock cubes, soy sauce and fish sauce) or at the point of consumption (e.g. table salt).

Salt intake can be reduced by:

- limiting the amount of salt and high-sodium condiments (e.g. soy sauce, fish sauce and bouillon) when cooking and preparing foods;
- not having salt or high-sodium sauces on the table;
- limiting the consumption of salty snacks; and
- choosing products with lower sodium content.

Some food manufacturers are reformulating recipes to reduce the sodium content of their products, and people should be encouraged to check nutrition labels to see how much sodium is in a product before purchasing or consuming it.

Potassium can mitigate the negative effects of elevated sodium consumption on blood pressure. Intake of potassium can be increased by consuming fresh fruit and vegetables.

Sugars

In both adults and children, the intake of free sugars should be reduced to less than 10% of total energy intake. A reduction to less than 5% of total energy intake would provide additional health benefits. Consuming free sugars increases the risk of dental caries (tooth decay). Excess calories from foods and drinks high in free sugars also contribute to unhealthy weight gain, which can lead to overweight and obesity. Recent evidence also shows that free sugars influence blood pressure and serum lipids, and suggests that a reduction in free sugars intake reduces risk factors for cardiovascular diseases (13).

Sugars intake can be reduced by:

- limiting the consumption of foods and drinks containing high amounts of sugars, such as sugary snacks, candies and sugar-sweetened beverages (i.e. all types of beverages containing free sugars – these include carbonated or non-carbonated soft drinks, fruit or vegetable juices and drinks, liquid and powder concentrates, flavored water, energy and sports drinks, ready-to-drink tea, ready-to-drink coffee and flavored milk drinks); and
- eating fresh fruit and raw vegetables as snacks instead of sugary snacks.

Reason why people follow a vegan diet

A vegan diet excludes all animal products—including meat, seafood, poultry, eggs and dairy products—and any foods with ingredients from an animal, like gelatin. Some vegans avoid honey too.

People choose to go vegan for environmental reasons, animal welfare and for the nutritional benefits of following a plant-based diet. According to the Humane Society International, eating a meat-free diet can cut our water footprint in half. Producing meat also creates more CO2 emissions and pollution than growing plants. And there's no denying that eating a plant-based diet is linked to longer life and reduced risk of chronic diseases like heart disease and cancer. Research shows that plant-based diets are low-cost, effective interventions for lowering body mass index, blood pressure, blood sugar (A1c) and cholesterol.

What is Keto diet

The keto (ketogenic) diet is a high-fat, moderate-protein, very-low-carbohydrate diet initially created in the 1920s for the treatment of epilepsy. Today, the keto diet has become a popular weight loss diet. When carbohydrate intake is extremely low, like on the keto diet, and the body's stores of glucose (glycogen) run out, the body begins to breakdown fat in the form of ketone bodies to provide energy. This is called ketosis and as long as carbohydrate intake is very low, and ketones are being used for fuel, the body will stay in this state of metabolism

Comparing keto diet and vegan diet

One diet is meat-heavy while the other eliminates all animal products. A vegan diet eliminates all animal products, while the keto diet strictly limits carbohydrates. There are no restrictions on calories or macronutrients on a vegan diet. The keto diet restricts carbohydrates in order to put your body into ketosis and convert the body's normal metabolism of glucose for energy to the metabolism of ketones for energy. There are technically no foods or food groups eliminated on keto. As long as you stick to about 80 percent of daily calories from fat, 15-20 percent from protein and less than 5 percent from carbohydrates, any foods are allowed. While a vegan diet is usually chosen for nutritional, ethical, religious and/or environmental reasons, the ketogenic diet is chosen for treatment of seizures, or more commonly nowadays, for weight loss.

Two popular diets — the vegan diet and the ketogenic diet — stand at polar opposites in terms of food strategy, but they're likewise popular for their promise to get the pounds off. Experts will tell you that you can expect to see results on either diet — but they may not last unless you can sustain this new lifestyle for the long term.

Many people on the keto diet do lose weight in the short run, but they also can lose mean muscle mass, and one study found they were no longer in ketosis six months after starting the diet.

For the vegan diet, one study found participants lost about 9 pounds over a year. But experts say that simply eating vegan doesn't guarantee weight loss, and similarly people may give up the diet due to it being very restrictive.

Similarities between vegan and keto

Both diets emphasize eating whole foods as much as possible, especially vegetables. But on keto you have to be careful with starchy vegetables like potatoes and corn, which could drive carb intake too high, depending on what else you're consuming that day.

Healthy fats are encouraged on both diets. The vegan diet recommends healthy fats to support overall health and wellbeing, while fat is the cornerstone of the keto diet, in order to keep the body in ketosis. However, because fat intake is so high on keto, many end up eating a lot of meat, cheese, butter and eggs—foods that are eliminated on a vegan diet. Plant-based sources of fat like olive oil, avocados, nuts and seeds are allowed on both diets.

Vegan and keto both encourage protein intake, but most keto dieters get protein from meat and dairy, while vegans may have a harder time getting enough protein in their diets, since plant-based proteins usually contain less protein per serving than animal products. The best protein sources for vegans are beans, legumes, tofu, whole grains, nuts and seeds.

Best diet for your life style and goals keto diet or vegan diet?

The most important question to ask when deciding what type of diet to follow is: Is this sustainable for me? Can I keep eating like this for the long-term?

With the keto diet especially, you may see rapid weight loss while following it, but if you can't sustain following the diet, you'll most likely gain the weight back once you stop the diet. It also depends on the foods choices you're making. A double bacon cheeseburger (hold the bun) and a salmon dinner with cucumber avocado salad are both keto dinners, but the salmon plate would provide you with more beneficial nutrients.

Even if you don't follow it forever, any period of eating a plant-based or vegan diet, will most likely deliver benefits in terms of reduced risk for chronic diseases and healthy cholesterol, blood sugar and blood pressure levels. You can also feel good about doing your part to help the environment. Some people choose to go partially vegan, meaning they may eat mostly vegan at home but not when eating outside the home, where it can be difficult to be fully vegan when you aren't doing the cooking. You can also eat mostly healthy plant-based foods, like fruits, vegetables and whole grains or consume mostly refined grains and vegan cookies.

The best diet is the one we can maintain for life and is only one piece of a healthy lifestyle. People should aim to eat high-quality, nutritious whole foods, mostly plants (fruits and veggies), and avoid flours, sugars, trans fats, and processed foods (anything in a box). Everyone should try to be physically active, aiming for about two and a half hours of vigorous activity per week. For many people, a healthy lifestyle also means better stress management, and perhaps even therapy to address emotional issues that can lead to unhealthy eating patterns.

Experts Opinion

When it comes to parsing the benefits of the keto diet and the vegan diet, experts will tell you that you can expect to see results on either diet — but they may not last unless you can sustain this new lifestyle for the long term. It turns out that's the hardest part of picking a diet. "When you bring up the concept of which diet is more successful for weight loss, I would only label a diet successful if it is sustainable," said Ashley Chambers, RD, a dietitian with Indiana University Health.

"Most diet trends for weight loss, such as the ketogenic diet and vegan diets, will lead to weight loss if you follow them strictly, but they often restrict so much that people have a hard time sustaining them for the long term." Dr. Charlie Seltzer, a Philadelphia-based, board-certified physician in obesity medicine and a clinical exercise specialist, agrees.

"You can only look at the success of a program if you're able to follow it," said Seltzer, who specializes in weight loss, lifestyle, and fitness solutions. "If it's unmaintainable over the long run, it doesn't really matter which is theoretically better." Seltzer says many people can try the keto diet and expect to see some success in the beginning.

However, he adds that the people you see posting their weight loss results on social media are the tip of the keto iceberg, as it were. They're the ones who've found a plan that works for them. That doesn't show you the multitude of people who haven't found success with the diet. "For every 100 people who try it, probably 99 of them will fail," Seltzer said. "That's because you can't do either of them for the rest of your life. They're difficult to do."

For Kristin Koskinen, RDN, who has a private practice in Washington State, the problem with the keto diet is what you're not eating. "My concern about keto is the long-term issues that may arise from limiting carbohydrates, which ultimately means plant-based foods," Koskinen said.

"My recommendation is that keto be used as a therapeutic tool or as a limited-duration strategy for weight loss. If you have diabetes or any other known health condition, consult with your healthcare provider before starting a keto diet."

That doesn't mean, however, that Koskinen falls in the vegan camp for weight loss either. "Though a vegan diet can be part of a healthy lifestyle, it doesn't always produce weight loss results," Koskinen said. "In my experience, choosing a vegan diet must accompany other lifestyle habits for weight loss, such as stress management and regular activity.

References

- Healthy diet. Geneva: World Health Organization; 2015 (Fact sheet No. 394; http://www.who.int/mediacentre/factsheets/fs394/en/,
- Adamsson V, Reumark A, Fredriksson IB, Hammarström E, Vessby B, Johansson G et al. Effects of a healthy Nordic diet on cardiovascular risk factors in hypercholesterolaemic subjects: a randomized controlled trial (NORDIET). J Intern Med. 2011;269(2):150–9.
- Kanerva N, Kaartinen NE, Rissanen H, Knekt P, Eriksson JG, Saaksjarvi K et al. Associations of the Baltic Sea diet with cardiometabolic risk factors: a meta-analysis of three Finnish studies. Br J Nutr. 2014;112(4):616–26.
- Lacoppidan SA, Kyrø C, Loft S, Helnæs A, Christensen J, Hansen CP et al. Adherence to a healthy Nordic food index is associated with a lower risk of type-2 diabetes: the Danish Diet, Cancer and Health Cohort Study. Nutrients. 2015;7(10):8633–44.
- Poulsen SK, Due A, Jordy AB, Kiens B, Stark KD, Stender S et al. Health effect of the New Nordic Diet in adults with increased waist circumference: a 6-mo randomized controlled trial. Am J Clin Nutr. 2014;99(1):35–45.
- About Health 2020. Copenhagen: WHO Regional Office for Europe; 2017 (http://www.euro.who.int/en/health-topics/health-policy/health-2020-the-europeanpolicy-for-health-and-well-being/about-health-2020, accessed 10 November 2017).
- European food and nutrition action plan 2015–2020. Copenhagen; WHO Regional Office for Europe; 2014 (EUR/RC64/R7).
- Salas-Salvadó J, Bulló M, Babio N, Martínez-González MÁ, Ibarrola-Jurado N, Basora J et al. Reduction in the incidence of type 2 diabetes with the Mediterranean diet. Results of the PREDIMED-Reus nutrition intervention randomized trial. Diabetes Care. 2011;34(1):14–19.

- Mediterranean diet pyramid: a lifestyle for today. Barcelona: Mediterranean Diet Foundation; 2017 (https://dietamediterranea.com/en/nutrition/, accessed 12 December 2017).
- Mediterranean diet: Cyprus, Croatia, Spain, Greece, Italy, Morocco and Portugal. Inscribed in 2013 (8.COM) on the Representative List of the Intangible Cultural Heritage of Humanity. Paris: United Nations Educational, Scientific and Cultural Organization; 2017 (http://www.unesco.org/culture/ich/en/RL/ mediterranean-diet-00884, accessed 10 November 2017).
- Schwingshackl L, Hoffmann G. Adherence to Mediterranean diet and risk of cancer: an updated systematic review and meta-analysis of observational studies. Cancer Med. 2015;4(12):1933–47.
- Singh B, Parsaik AK, Mielke MM, Erwin PJ, Knopman DS, Petersen RC et al. Association of Mediterranean diet with mild cognitive impairment and Alzheimer's disease: a systematic review and meta-analysis. J Alzheimers Dis. 2014;39(2):271–82.
- Grosso G, Mistretta A, Frigiola A, Gruttadauria S, Biondi A, Basile F et al. Mediterranean diet and cardiovascular risk factors: a systematic review. Crit Rev Food Sci Nutr. 2014;54(5):593–610. 40.
- García-Fernández E, Rico-Cabanas L, Rosgaard N, Estruch R, Bach-Faig A. Mediterranean diet and cardio diabesity: a review. Nutrients. 2014;6(9):3474.
- GBD Compare. In: Institute for Health Metrics and Evaluation [website]. Seattle (WA): University of Washington; 2016 (http://vizhub.healthdata.org/ gbd-compare, accessed 6 December 2016
- 41. Gonzalez CA, Riboli E. Diet and cancer prevention: contributions from the European Prospective Investigation into Cancer and Nutrition (EPIC) study. Eur J Cancer. 2010;46(14):2555–62.
- Alcalay RN, Gu Y, Mejia-Santana H, Cote L, Marder KS, Scarmeas N. The association between Mediterranean diet adherence and Parkinson's disease. Mov Disord. 2012;27(6):771–4.

- Estruch R, Ros E, Salas-Salvadó J, Covas M-I, Corella D, Arós F et al. Primary prevention of cardiovascular disease with a Mediterranean diet. N Engl J Med. 2013;368(14):1279–90.
- Krauss RM, Eckel RH, Howard B, Appel LJ, Daniels SR, Deckelbaum RJ et al. AHA dietary guidelines: revision 2000 – a statement for healthcare professionals from the Nutrition Committee of the American Heart Association. Circulation. 2000;102(18):2284–99.
- Keys A, Menotti A, Karvonen MJ, Aravanis C, Blackburn H, Buzina R et al. The diet and 15-year death rate in the seven countries study. Am J Epidemiol. 1986;124(6):903–15.
- Tong TYN, Wareham NJ, Khaw K-T, Imamura F, Forouhi NG. Prospective association of the Mediterranean diet with cardiovascular disease incidence and mortality and its population impact in a non-Mediterranean population: the EPIC–Norfolk study. BMC Med. 2016;14(1):135
- Esposito K, Maiorino MI, Ceriello A, Giugliano D. Prevention and control of type 2 diabetes by Mediterranean diet: a systematic review. Diabetes Res Clin Pract. 2010;89(2):97–102.
- Esposito K, Maiorino MI, Ciotola M, Di Palo C, Scognamiglio P, Gicchino M et al. Effects of a Mediterranean-style diet on the need for antihyperglycemic drug therapy in patients with newly diagnosed type 2 diabetes: a randomized trial. Ann Intern Med. 2009;151(5):306–14.
- Shai I, Schwarzfuchs D, Henkin Y, Shahar DR, Witkow S, Greenberg I et al. Weight loss with a low-carbohydrate, Mediterranean, or low-fat diet. N Engl J Med. 2008;359(3):229–41.
- Sofi F, Cesari F, Abbate R, Gensini GF, Casini A. Adherence to Mediterranean diet and health status: meta-analysis. BMJ. 2008;337:a1344.
- Noncommunicable diseases progress monitor. Geneva: World Health Organization; 2015
- World report on ageing and health. Geneva: World Health Organization; 2015.
- Migration and health: key issues. Copenhagen: WHO Regional Office for Europe; 2017 (http://www.euro.who.int/en/health-topics/health-determinants/ migration-and-health/migrant-

- health-in-the-european-region/migrationand-health-key-issues, accessed 3 June 2017).
- Watts N, Adger WN, Agnolucci P, Blackstock J, Byass P, Cai W et al. Health and climate change: policy responses to protect public health. Lancet. 386(10006):1861–914.
- Friel S, Bowen K, Campbell-Lendrum D, Frumkin H, McMichael AJ, Rasanathan K. Climate change, noncommunicable diseases, and development: the relationships and common policy opportunities. Annu Rev Public Health. 2011;32:133–47.
- The UN decade of action on nutrition. New York: United Nations System Standing Committee on Nutrition; 2016 (https://www.unscn.org/en/topics/ un-decade-of-action-on-nutrition, accessed 26 February 2018).
- Gushulak B, Weekers J, Macpherson D. Migrants and emerging public health issues in a globalized world: threats, risks and challenges, an evidence-based framework. Emerg Health Threats J. 2009;2:e10.
- Serra-Majem L, Aranceta J, SENC Working Group. Guía de la alimentación saludable [The healthy food guide]. Madrid: Spanish Society of Community Nutrition; 2004.
- Drake I, Gullberg B, Ericson U, Sonestedt E, Nilsson J et al. Development of a diet quality index assessing adherence to the Swedish nutrition recommendations and dietary guidelines in the Malmö diet and cancer cohort. Public Health Nutr. 2011;14(5):835–45.
- Come sano y muévete: 12 decisiones saludables [Eat healthy and move: 12 healthy choices]. Madrid: Spanish Agency for Food Safety and Nutrition; 2008 (in Spanish).
- Hlebowicz J, Drake I, Gullberg B, Sonestedt E, Wallström P, Persson M et al. A high diet quality is associated with lower incidence of cardiovascular events in the Malmö diet and cancer cohort. PLOS ONE. 2013;8(8):e71095
- Appel, L. J., Moore, T. J., Obarzanek, E., Vollmer, W. M., Svetkey, L. P., Sacks, F. M., … Karanja, N. (1997). A clinical trial of the effects of dietary patterns on blood pressure, The New England Journal of Medicine, 336(16), 1117–1124. https:// doi: 10.1056/NEJM199704173361601 Appleton, K. M., Rogers, P. J., & Ness, A. R. (2010). Updated systematic review and meta-analysis of the effects of n–3 long-chain polyunsaturated fatty

acids on depressed mood. The American Journal of Clinical Nutrition, 91(3), 757–770. https://doi.org/10.3945/ajcn.2009.28313

- Aridi, Y. S., Walker, J. L., & Wright, O. R. L. (2017). The association between the Mediterranean dietary pattern and cognitive health: A systematic review. Nutrients, 9(674), 1–23. https://doi.org/10.3390/nu9070674

- ATBC Cancer Prevention Study Group. (1994). The alpha-tocopherol, beta-carotene lung cancer prevention study: Design, methods, participant characteristics, and compliance. Annals of Epidemiology, 4(1), 1–10. https://doi.org/10.106/1047-2797(94)90036-1

- Bach-Faig, A., Berry, E. M., Lairon, D., Reguant, J., Trichopoulou, A., Dernini, S., … Padulosi, S. (2011). Mediterranean diet pyramid today. Science and cultural updates. Public Health Nutrition, 14(12A), 2274–2284. https://doi.org/10.1017/S1368980011002515

- Marx, W., Moseley, G., Berk, M., & Jacka, F. (2017). Nutritional psychiatry: the present state of the evidence. Proceedings of the Nutrition Society, 76(04), 427–436. https://doi.org/10.1017/s0029665117002026

- Mayer, E. A., Knight, R., Mazmanian, S. K., Cryan, J. F., & Tillisch, K. (2014). Gut Microbes and the Brain: Paradigm Shift in Neuroscience. Journal of Neuroscience, 34(46), 15490– 15496. https://doi.org/10.1523/JNEUROSCI.3299-14.2014

- Wärnberg, J., Gomez-Martinez, S., Romeo, J., Díaz, L. E., & Marcos, A. (2009). Nutrition, inflammation, and cognitive function. In Annals of the New York Academy of Sciences. https://doi.org/10.1111/j.1749-6632.2008.03985.x Scientific Reports, 7, 1–9. https://doi.org/10.1038/srep41317

- Sánchez-Villegas, A., Martínez-González, M. A., Estruch, R., Salas-Salvadó, J., Corella, D., Covas, M. I., … Serra-Majem, L. (2013). Mediterranean dietary pattern and depression: the PREDIMED randomized trial. BMC Medicine, 11(1), 1–11. https://doi.org/10.1186/1741-7015-11-208

- Buettner, D. (2012, October 24). The Island Where People Forget to Die. Retrieved May 4, 2018, from https://www.nytimes.com/2012/10/28/magazine/the-isalnd-where-people-forget-to-die.html?_r=0

- The Blue Zones Story. (n.d.). Retrieved May 4, 2018, from https://www.bluezones.com/
- Barclay, E. (2015, April 11). Eating To Break 100: Longevity Diet Tips From The Blue Zones. Retrieved May 4, 2018, from https://www.npr.org/sections/ththesalt/2015/04/11/398325030/eatings-to-break-100-longevity-diet-tips-from-the-blue-zones
- Volek, J.S., W.J. Kraemer, J.A. Bush, T. Incledon, and M. Boetes. Testosterone and cortisol in relationship to dietary nutrients and resistance exercise. J. Appl. Physiol. 82(1):49-54. 1997
- Economos, C.D., S.S. Bortz, and M.E. Nelson. Nutritional practices of elite athletes: Practical recommendations. Sports Med. 16(6):381-399. 1993.
- Wheeler, K. Proteins and amino acids. NSCA Journal. 10(6):22,28-29. 1988.
- Ellis, D., and K. Gabel. Weight gain guidelines for athletes. NSCA Journal. 13(3):20-23. 1991.
- Walberg-Rankin, J. A review of nutritional practices and needs of bodybuilders. J. Strength and Cond. Res. 9(2):116-124. 1995.
- http://www.womenrunning.com/health/food-help-balance-hormones/
- (Serra-Majem L, Aranceta J, SENC Working Group. Guía de la alimentación saludable [The healthy food guide]. Madrid: Spanish Society of Community Nutrition; 2004.),